CUMBRIA LIBRARIES
38003050706...
KT-491-371

Clare and Greg Wise were born and raised in the north of England. She read books, he fell out of trees. She excelled at school, he hid when the end-of-term report came. She got a double first in history at university. He did two degrees – one where you spend your time drawing (architecture), the other where you pretend to be someone else (acting).

As adults, they both found themselves in the film business: she originally at the UK Film Council and then a vice president at Universal Pictures, he still dressing up and pretending to be someone else.

They lived in the same street until her death in 2016.

'Inspirational'
Daily Mail

'A remarkable account of illness, loss and the power of sibling love'
The Times

'Wise's reflections on compassion fatigue are worth the price of this book alone, but what you take away is something splendid and unwearying: a sibling's devotion that feels remarkably like what we mean when we talk of a stage of grace'
Daily Telegraph

Not That Kind of Love

CLARE WISE AND GREG WISE

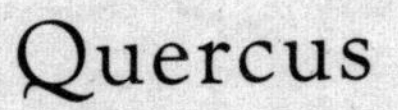
Quercus

First published in Great Britain in 2018 by Quercus Editions Ltd
This paperback edition published in 2018 by

Quercus Editions Ltd
Carmelite House
50 Victoria Embankment
London EC4Y 0DZ

An Hachette UK company

Copyright © 2018 Greg Wise

The moral right of Greg Wise to be
identified as the author of this work has been
asserted in accordance with the
Copyright, Designs and Patents Act, 1988.

All rights reserved. No part of this publication
may be reproduced or transmitted in any form
or by any means, electronic or mechanical,
including photocopy, recording, or any
information storage and retrieval system,
without permission in writing from the publisher.

A CIP catalogue record for this book is available
from the British Library

ISBN 978 1 78648 896 1

Every effort has been made to contact copyright holders.
However, the publishers will be glad to rectify in future editions
any inadvertentomissions brought to their attention.

Quercus Editions Ltd hereby exclude all liability to the extent permittedby law
for any errors or omissions in this book and for any loss, damage or expense
(whether direct or indirect) suffered by a third party relying on
any information contained in this book.

CREDITS

Line illustrations by Paul Thomas
Portraits of Clare, pages 50 and 54, by Tina Ninua
Photographs: pages 31, 49, 50, 128, 283 and 287 by Richard Jinman;
p. 91: Copyright © WENN Ltd/Alamy Stock Photo; p.99: Copyright
© Charlotte Murphy; p.100: Copyright © Getty Images/Dave M.
Benett; Front cover, inside cover and pages 243, 291 by Rose Smith;
p.278: Copyright © Michael Chambati-Woodhead; p.234: Copyright
© Nick Wall; All other photographs are the authors' own
Text credit: 'Hope for the Terminally Ill' article quoted on page 273:
copyright © 2000, BMJ Publishing Group Ltd

10 9 8 7 6 5 4 3 2

Typeset in Harriet Text by Lindsay Nash
Printed and bound in Great Britain by Clays Ltd, Elcograf S.p.A.

Not That Kind of Love

Some or all of this may be true:

I gave up my career as an international spy to take cover in the world of film. For a long time (a quarter of a century... doesn't that sound impressive?) I worked as a film producer/executive/dogsbody and had a great, albeit often stressful, time. Then in 2013 I got cancer... possibly the two are related... anyway, I started this blog so that my friends and distant family wouldn't have to keep asking me about my health. To my great surprise I found out that I really loved blogging, and so when the cancer returned with a vengeance this year, I decided to carry on.

As I write this section in November 2015 I have had 96,000 hits on the site and messages and comments from all over the world, many from people I don't know. It's been a wonderful experience (cancer aside) and it has spurred me on to think about writing other things. Apart from spying, my other great passion is travelling, and luckily the two coalesced and I am starting to write a book on snapshots from around the world. I aim to get it finished before I slip off this mortal coil.

Clare x

Where do you want the blind hanging?

27 MAY 2013

'Go home and prepare for the worst' – no one but Morgan Freeman as the US President should ever say this unless a meteorite is about to hit the Earth and neither Will Smith nor Bruce Willis is available to save us.

But this was said to me on 7 May 2013... WHAT DOES IT MEAN?

I need to start this blog with a bit of history. I apologize for my verbosity. My English teacher at school used to scold me by saying 'less verbosity, more pith'... but his name was 'Rosie' Bullcock so we can pretty much ignore him. Suffice it to say there's a reason I don't have a Twitter account, apart from not understanding how I can condense what I need to say into 142 characters or whatever it is.

I found my first lump in 2007. When I say 'found', this is a bit of an exaggeration. I guess the truth is I couldn't really miss it. I don't have a close relationship with my body. It is more like that of a third cousin several times removed – the one you only ever see when your second cousin several times removed organizes some sort of family get-together.

I know people, women in particular, who are so in tune with their own bodies that they can tell when they are ovulating or growing a nail. I never even heard or felt my PMT until after the event. So to say I 'found' a lump is really untrue.

I was in Beijing – my least-favourite city. On the whole I love travelling and I love hotels. I even loved this hotel in Beijing. The only issue I have with all hotel architects and designers is that they insist on putting so many mirrors in the bathroom that you can see your cellulite from every angle multiplied into infinity. This is amplified by the lighting in hotel bathrooms, which is ideal if you want to pluck your moustache or eyebrows but awful if you want to ignore your wrinkles, worry lines, stretch marks or any other imperfection.

In this bathroom what I saw was something protruding from my breast. It was sort of torpedo-shaped – very like the plastic thing inside a Kinder egg which holds the disappointingly fragile toy.

Of course I expected it to go away.

It didn't, and by the time I got home it was hot, very hot, and anything in contact with it was painful. Since going to work topless was not an option (I worked for a government quango and there are rules about such things), I went to my GP.

I have been with my surgery for over twenty years. In all that time I have never seen the same GP twice. The surgery is in a poor part of London and the catchment area is huge. It is on what we commonly call the Kilburn Thyroid – but which is actually called the Kilburn High Road. Traditionally an Irish area, it is now as multicultural as the rest of London and the surgery has to reflect this diversity.

The other thing about the surgery is that they seem to have an unwritten policy of not spending more than three minutes with each patient.

There's a famous agent in Hollywood called Robert Newman, previously of ICM and now of WME. His meetings last for no more than two minutes sixteen seconds, unless of course you are a client and have made the firm lots of money. Two minutes sixteen seconds is just enough time to enter the room, stretch out your hand for a handshake and introduce yourself, look for somewhere to perch (he has one of those adjustable-height desks set at thorax height so he doesn't have to waste time sitting down) and then struggle to take off your jacket, pitch your idea, put your jacket back on and leave . . . that's two minutes sixteen seconds later.

It's like that at my GP surgery. Until this time. When the lady GP in the headscarf saw my lump, she had to make a call to the local hospital and what with the automatic answering and the 'press one if your call is urgent and you are bleeding to death and two if you don't mind waiting for hours in A & E', I think I was there for two patient slots – about five minutes.

I asked my brother to come to the hospital with me. Greg is great in A & E – partly because he can juggle (and make balloon animals but needs some prior warning to bring all the kit) but mostly because he is funny and charming and virtually every nurse in every hospital either recognizes him or goes into flirt overdrive.

Luckily it was a Wednesday afternoon so it wasn't full of Friday-night casualties. It was the usual collection of A & E stalwarts.

Every time I go to A & E it seems that you have to have the following in order to qualify for your NHS status: a builder covered in plaster dust carrying his arm or hand in a bloodied workcloth; a cycle courier with a hole in the spandex round about the knee; a small boy in some kind of sports gear; a man in a dodgy-looking leisure suit with a gold chain on the phone in some sort of Slavic language; and a girl in Ugg boots and skin-tight jeggings, hobbling.

But a breast lump allows you to jump the queue.

After filling in paperwork and every nurse in the building 'popping by' to see Greg, a young chap appeared in a white coat. He was a sallow youth. Still had teenage acne, glasses and probably halitosis, but I wasn't going to check.

'Hello, I'm from the breast clinic. I am here to examine you.'

Whereupon Greg said (as would anyone of us), 'I bet you say that to all the girls and you're really a heating engineer.'

This poor boy went several shades that Farrow & Ball make (a posh painting company, for the non-English, non-middle-class DIY enthusiasts amongst you) and then Greg and I spent ages talking him down, telling him jokes and things to make him feel better. Like the one about the mother superior taking a bath in the convent when there's a knock at the door.

'It's the blind man from the village, can I come in?'

'Yes, enter.'

'Nice tits. Where do you want the blind hanging?'

The upshot of all this was that I have what is called in the medical profession 'lumpy breasts'. Prosaic. They are also called 'breast mice' and are little fibroid adenomas which occasionally become infected and have to be aspirated. Basically, though, they have always been benign.

The second time it happened was two years later and I was referred to the breast clinic at University College Hospital (UCH) where I had my first mammogram. I know that every woman who has ever had one will tell you that the first thing they say after experiencing it is, 'I bet that was designed by a man.' It was indeed a man – Albert Salomon. It is an excruciating procedure but better than waiting until the cancer is so advanced they can see it in surgery and you die anyway.

Imagine, if you will, one of those Builders' Mate's vices that you see advertised around bank holiday weekends when the weather will be shit and all the menfolk will be able to do is craft something in their garages.

You have to fit your very sensitive breasts (think testicles, chaps) onto a cold glass plate and then another plate squashes it down until it's virtually flat (not what nature intended) and then hold it there for forty-five seconds. You do this horizontally and then vertically on each breast. There are no expletives strong enough to cover the pain.

The worst thing is that I not only have breast mice (and no breast cat) but I also have 'dense' breasts. OMG, on top of lumpy mammaries I now have stupid breasts. In defence, I would like to say that I have gorgeous tits. An artist wanted to cast them in bronze and even at this advanced age I can still go bra-less without having to tuck them into the waistband of my jeans.

So I became used to lumps, mammograms and all that my stupid breasts want to throw at me. Until three weeks ago.

Six weeks ago I got another one of my Kinder-egg, torpedo lumps and tried to go direct to the breast clinic but they wanted a GP referral. Back to the Thyroid, sit in waiting room with Somalis, Afghans, Africans, Russians, Bosnians and pretty much every other nationality on the planet. My doctor this time was Egyptian. He referred me to the clinic for three weeks hence.

I went to the US – had a great road trip around Arizona and California (more on this later) and came back to an appointment at the new Macmillan Cancer Centre at UCH.

I knew conclusively that I didn't have cancer and this was just a precaution as the breast clinic had been moved there. After three and a half hours of ultrasounds, mammograms, aspirations, biopsies and being shadowed by a male nurse who looked distinctly peaky when the large needle (size of a Hobbit's spear) was being inserted into my breast... I finally went into a room where I was outnumbered five to one by nurses and specialists. This is when I was told that they were 'ninety-five per cent' sure I had cancer and to 'go home and prepare for the worst and come back in seven days for the diagnosis'.

WTF???? How can you be 95 per cent sure and how can I go home for a week and prepare for the worst... what does that mean? Do I go to Sainsbury's and buy bottled water? Stock up on cat food? Wander the streets looking like Munch's *The Scream*? What do I do? Vodka seemed a sensible option... so I pretty much spent all of that week inebriated.

A week later I took Greg (for all the aforementioned reasons) and after waiting for over an hour (that's a whole week and an hour of preparing for the worst) it was confirmed. I have a 3.5-centimetre tumour in my left breast and cells in my lymph nodes of the left armpit.

The weird thing is that the second someone tells you that you have cancer your brain goes into cloud cuckoo land. There was no way that I could tell you exactly what my oncoplastic surgeon said to me – when I saw that her mouth had stopped moving and she asked me if I had any questions all that I could think of was, 'Where did you get your dress?' After she explained I would start chemo very shortly, etc. etc., and that I would have to have an MRI, a CT scan, bone scan, etc. etc... did I have any other questions? To which I answered, 'Can I have it done on a beach in Mauritius?'

I am clearly a cancer moron.

But as my senior oncologist said to me, 'We are not treating your IQ, we are treating your cancer.' Phew! Dodged that bullet then.

Will I grow a beard?

31 MAY 2013

The thing is I don't feel ill or sick but everyone I talk to in the medical profession is telling me that I will feel sick after 6 June, when the chemo starts. That's a very strange concept – a pre-warning of illness. Ironically, apart from all the holes in me from needles and biopsies, I feel great. I don't feel depressed and I don't feel like I might need to cry. What's there to cry about at the moment? None of this feels real. In fact, what I have is theoretical cancer which will be treated by theoretical chemotherapy starting 6 June and theoretical surgery in November and possible radiotherapy thereafter. I will theoretically go bald, my nails may fall out, the soles of my feet and the palms of my hands will go red, my ankles will swell and I will be nauseous with a mouth full of ulcers, no taste buds and itchy skin. Hurrah.

Cancer appears to have been identified in the fourth century BC by Hippocrates (he of the oath) and he named the appearance of the tumours as '*Carcinos*' which means crab or crayfish in Greek. Typical – I am allergic to shellfish…

The poor cancer sufferers in the intervening twenty-three centuries had horrible treatments with little or no success. The Egyptians, of course, had discovered breast cancer in 1600 BC and would cauterize the tumours, but that wasn't a cure.

(At this point I would like to thank the marvellous Interweb for giving me some of the facts and a rather scary book called *Coping with Chemotherapy* which someone sent me. They should remain anonymous as really what I need is a book called *Not Coping with Theoretical Chemotherapy* – either that or lots of chocolate and/or alcohol whilst I can still taste it.)

Chemotherapy wasn't developed until the mid-twentieth century when two American doctors treating veterans of the First World War mustard-gas attacks discovered that by injecting the ex-soldiers who had developed leukaemia or lymphomas with the mustine chemical they could treat the cancer. And thus it was that doses of toxic poison were developed and refined and given very complicated names with horrible side effects and bundled under the term chemotherapy.

Obviously the great Marie Curie's invention of radiation has revolutionized the treatment and diagnosis of cancer, but ultimately the patient still has to find a lump, or notice a change in their body or be dissected after death for cancer to be discovered in them.

Enough of this serious stuff and back to my stupid mouse-infested breasts.

Straight after diagnosis the NHS went into a frenzy of tests on me. The first was an MRI. A truly magnificent piece of equipment – once assembled in a hospital it can't be moved after it is built in situ. It's basically a gigantic magnet which emits waves and stuff. If it was outside, the closest anyone could get to it when it was on would be to stand on the far side of the next block, or as the nurse cheerfully said whilst strapping me in, 'about the length of a large Sainsbury's car park away'.

The walls and ceilings and floors and doors around an MRI scanner are several feet thick and once you've been manoeuvred into place, strapped down and injected with dye, the lab assistants and radiologists retreat into rooms literally on the other side of the building. That's the easy part. If you have any piercings ('internal as well as external', according to my nurse) you have to take them off as they will be whipped off into the magnet.

Because they were looking at my torso I had to lie face down with my poor breasts squashed into square metal boxes which tightened around them (there's a theme building here) and lie in the tube for forty minutes. The machine makes a terrible din. Think of the soundtrack of *Die Another Day* on steroids with you sitting under five speakers at Dobly 11 (and yes, I do mean that spelling, in homage to the 1984 mockumentary *This Is Spinal Tap*...) in the Empire Leicester Square. There are headphones provided by the NHS so the radiologist (who by now is in a Starbucks round the corner on a laptop) can talk to you. They are not those very expensive noise-reducing headphones that you are tempted by in the British Airways Duty Free catalogue or indeed Dr Dre Beats – they are more like they were nicked from a long-haul BA flight when the wearer in economy had got bored and chewed off the spongy bit.

However, to soothe you, you are offered music... modern, ballads, techno? Really? Not me. Classical... OK, give that a shot. I swear I was given Wagner's *Ring Cycle* and halfway through the scan, when this belting soprano was about to throw herself off something or into something, both the machine and the music built to such a crescendo I could feel my heart beating so loudly and fast that I thought it might explode... This, combined with the deafening magnety noise and the claustrophobia, and I did start to feel as though waterboarding at Glyndebourne might be preferable. I am not sure that they offer this yet.

After the MRI scan I went back to the Cancer Centre and had another biopsy. A Hobbit's sword of a needle going into my other breast was pure heaven in comparison. This biopsy was much more complicated, though, as the mice on the right side, presumably having got word from the inhabitants on the left side, decided to quite literally play cat and mouse. My poor ultrasound radiologist specialist had to chase them all through the dense tissue of the breast. Three different places and three different attempts. Ouch.

The next scan was a CT scan – don't worry, this will be easy in comparison, I was told. Easy, my foot. You can't eat for six hours before the scan. Mine was an afternoon appointment. I had asked a friend to pal me for this. She quite sensibly booked lunch at a gorgeous restaurant nearby. I didn't read the letter about the scan until I was en route to lunch. Nil by mouth... what? Shall we cancel...? Too late. So instead I sat and watched her eat a rather delicious-looking lunch. (This cancer thing just gets better and better.) Very sweetly, though, she ordered a shellfish pasta which I wouldn't have been able to eat anyway and decided not to order a dessert as that would have been cruel.

The scan was in the basement of the Cancer Centre. It was us and four blokes. We all had to sit in a very small corridor in our hospital gowns without anything on bar our knickers and socks. I was as uncomfortable as they were. My friend tried to make me feel more at ease by taking the mickey out of my socks. Basically, I have lots of airline socks and nothing else. I flew a lot when I was still gainfully employed and I couldn't resist an airline sock, especially Virgin Atlantic. So there I was sitting in an ill-fitting gown (you know the ones that tie at the back but which seem to have lost at least one of the ties...) and my socks which say VIRGIN on the base – the ATLANTIC must have washed off.

The CT machine is a giant rotating magnetic coil. You are given three different lots of dye, injected into your veins by the machine during the scan. The first one makes you feel very hot and like you've wet yourself. Nice. So a badly fitting gown, airline socks, four blokes sitting outside the cubicle you have to use to change, and a wet patch. Going bald will seem like a walk in the park after this.

Actually, you don't wee. But you feel like you have. You also have to hold your breath whilst this giant doughnut of metal whirrs around you. I didn't like that one. It was better than the MRI but the waterboarding was still looking good.

My most recent scan was yesterday. A bone scan at the department of nuclear medicine. That's enough to make you draw breath. You have to have an injection three hours before the scan. They inject you with radioactive material. Then you go off and have to drink at least two litres of water, come back, pee and then lie in another machine for thirty minutes. I really need to start reading the accompanying material when I go to these things – it wasn't until this morning that I realized that last night I should have drunk another two litres of water. I did drink a lot of fluid but it was French and red and in a green bottle. They also don't tell you that your pee turns fluorescent green. What they do tell you is you could set off X-ray and security machines at airports for up to twenty-four hours afterwards. Sadly, I couldn't find anywhere to travel to last night.

What made the whole experience even more surreal was that a friend came with me and during the scan did Reiki on me... holding first my feet and then my head. Once again you are strapped onto a metal slide (this time by a lovely Indian nurse from Kerala who recommended taking a rice boat) and a large flat metal plate is put above and around you. It is marked with a cross hair that travels very slowly along all of your body photographing the insides of your bones. So I had the cross hair above me and John at my feet telling me to notice my breath. Notice my breath... I was so busy concentrating on avoiding the sniper I could barely breathe.

Apart from the scans I have also met the oncology team and the wig maker. The last one should really be the title of a John Grisham novel... she was the wig maker with the worst dye job ever. It reminded me of when I chaired a BAFTA jury on Hair and Make-Up and had twelve of the leading specialists in the field (not nominated in that year) as the jury. I'm not sure I have seen worse hair and make-up in one room. Next time I will get drag queens.

The NHS wigs are made from synthetic hair. You choose three different styles from a catalogue and then three different colours. The styles are all called by women's names – I chose a Lexy, an Angela and a Claire. They are all very over-layered and all two-tone (highlights), not quite Farrah Fawcett-Majors – if you decide to buy one you can restyle it at home (a recipe for disaster if there was ever one . . . I only ever cut my fringe drunk late at night and regret it in the morning and hope it will grow out soon).

My oncology team are lovely. The registrar and the oncologist are both beautiful women. I think one is Persian and the other Indian. They are slim, well groomed, with gorgeous skin, long flowing healthy hair and basically perfect. They tell you (repeatedly) that you will swell up with the steroids, get fat ankles, lose your hair everywhere apart from your legs, have red palms and feet, constant diarrhoea and feel sick. I think the team need to rethink this approach and hire one of those dwarves from *The Lord of the Rings* who is ugly and squat to deliver this message. It would be easier to handle if you could feel superior to the purveyor of such news.

My hair may grow back curly and possibly grey or silver – the same colour as the senior oncologist's hair.

He also has a beard. When he told me my hair might grow back like his I got confused – will I also grow a beard? He is hopeful because then he could write an award-winning paper about me.

I will see what I can do.

Handy tips

2 JUNE 2013

I saw a book last week called *Crafts with Your Cat's Hair* – it was an entire book about what to make with the fur balls from your cat. I am tempted to launch one called *Crafts with Your Own Hair* – just imagine what finger puppets, pincushions, Christmas ornaments I could make with my Titian locks. I may ask Steven my hairdresser to keep the longer bits so I can experiment with knitting them.

Sadly, the hair is not long enough to make a wig from so I can't recycle my own hair that way, but watch this space for a range of inexpensive Christmas presents.

On my twenty-first birthday I was in London with my father. He was presenting a conference in the Docklands at a TV studio there and in the next studio were the offices and sets for *Spitting Image*. I had much longer hair then and Prince Andrew had just got engaged or married to Sarah Ferguson. I was approached in the loo by a lady brandishing scissors who offered to give me a free haircut in exchange for my hair for the Fergie puppet. Too good an offer for a poor student to refuse. They also gave me some cash, which was later taken from me in my only experience of being mugged in London. Oh well, you win some, you lose some.

There are so many tips for someone about to go through chemo, getting through chemo and recovering from chemo. There are the obvious diet ones, of course, as well as diets that you should have followed so you wouldn't get cancer in the first place. The one that appeals most to me is to have a treat a day. If anyone out there has any suggestions do let me know. Think of it as an unbucket list. I am not yet ready to do the BIG list where I pretend I really want to skydive or swim with sharks before I die... no, this is a gentler home-based list. Things like, have a square of chocolate, paint on false eyebrows, pluck your hairy legs... that kind of thing.

Eating tips also gratefully received. I am told that a little glass of dry sherry helps with nausea (it may well cause nausea in me as I am not nearly old enough to have a dry sherry each day, but on the other hand I do have a selection of turbans so maybe I am middle-aged). Another tip for nausea is to drink sodium bicarbonate... the sherry looks good right about now. Green tea, of course, is a must, as are leafy green veg, oily fish and cutting out dairy and salt. I am going to be the most boring guest – the ones you dread coming round as they are intolerant to everything.

The clock is ticking and I am trying not to drink alcohol again before Thursday. Mostly because I have to have my blood, liver and kidneys tested and I don't want to be reminded that I am an overweight alcoholic. For those of you who don't know this yet, I rather foolishly agreed to a free health test on the NHS this time last year. Naively I thought it would be one of those intensive BUPA tests where every organ is checked out. Hmmm. No, this is Austerity Britain. A rather dumpy nurse measured me, weighed me and took a pinprick of blood to test for diabetes. She asked me to describe my diet and alcohol intake so I did what any self-respecting person does – I halved my alcohol intake for the questionnaire. At the end of the consultation (a big word for five minutes with a nurse) she triumphantly informed me in the eyes of Camden NHS I am an 'overweight alcoholic' and I would now be offered diet counselling or addiction counselling. PLEASE.

Here's to a few days of clean living to prep for toxic meltdown. I will post photos of the new short hair and my wigs in the next few days. I have already borrowed a rather gorgeous brunette one. My niece is keen that I don't wear a beanie without a wig, unless I want to look like 'Care in the Community'. God forbid a bald, spotty, hairy-legged, red-palmed, swollen-ankled, sherry-drinking, middle-aged Clare would look like 'care in the community'. I will look more like an escaped Gruffalo.

D-Day

3 JUNE 2013

This year on 6 June, sixty-nine years after the Allies stormed the Normandy beaches, my own defences will be stormed by a cocktail of toxic poisons. Yum yum.

It is somehow appropriate that it should all kick off on D-Day. I do feel as if I am waiting for a climactic event and there is only so much prep that I can do. I have bought several turbans – including a rather fancy black silk one with a Swarovski brooch for evening wear. I look like a cross between a 1950s housewife extolling the virtues of a wizard new cleaning product and Hilda Ogden. Stupidly, I had assumed I would look like Gloria Swanson. There is definitely a swansong here . . . I should have followed Steph's advice and allowed myself to be styled by a drag artiste. It's not too late. Steph, for those of you who don't know, wrote and directed the hit film *The Adventures of Priscilla, Queen of the Desert*.

There are so many websites offering chemo-specific headgear. Most of them are scary. I could end up looking like a pirate, and not Johnny Depp . . . one of the ugly extras. Greg thinks I should opt for the full burka. It's a thought and one I haven't yet fully dismissed. I did get a couple of beanies. They really are awful things and I look like I have put a tea cosy on my head. There must be a better solution.

On a brighter note my synthetic two-tone wigs have arrived and I will try them on at the hospital on D-Day minus one when I have to go for a pre-chemo check. I guess it's like when you join a gym and some nice buffed Kiwi man with large arm muscles and an impossibly small waist shows you all the machines and you try to look like you will be using them regularly. I expect I will be shown around the chemo floor of the hospital. And like at the gym they will want to weigh and measure me. But unlike the gym they also want blood from me. I really need to keep track about the number of needles I have had stuck into me. It might make for a good stat.

The Cancer Centre is magnificent and would definitely be worth a visit if it weren't for all the sick people which might put off the tourists. It is a brand new five-storey building. The atrium has a huge mobile hanging over the reception desk. It is called *Strand* and is by an artist who walked all the beaches in England picking up bits of plastic detritus and hung them very tastefully in a vast mobile. Last week one of the bits of plastic fell off, injuring a receptionist, so the desk has been shut down by Health and Safety.

I was in there yesterday and for the first time I noticed sick people. I don't know whether when you first get diagnosed they hide the sick from you so as not to frighten you or whether it depends on the day – apparently chemo for breast cancer is always done on a Thursday – but whatever the reason the place was full of bald, bewigged, sick people. One in particular caught my eye. A car crash of styles. A Marilyn Monroe wig, baby-doll dress and tights – one leg green and one leg orange. I was just thinking to myself somewhat smugly that even on my worst Hobbity day I wouldn't look that bad when I realized it was Grayson Perry, the transvestite Turner Award-winning artist who has decorated the chemo floor. It's an encouraging sign when even the rich and famous want to look like they are dressed by the NHS wig and make-up department.

Talking of the rich and famous, I am in awe of Angelina Jolie – she has leapt in my estimation. Good on her for having the double mastectomy and letting the world know. That's very brave. I think I might get T-shirts printed for the staff at the hospital saying WHAT WOULD ANGIE DO? Or perhaps just shortened to WWAD?

I was on the Tube on the way home and by accident I had hit rush hour, which as you Londoners know is any time between 8 a.m. and 8 p.m., and found myself wedged between a smelly armpit and an *Evening Standard*. I really wanted a seat but none were free. London transport gives pregnant women badges that say BABY ON BOARD. I am going to write to them to see if they might make me one that says CANCER ON BOARD or even TUMOUR ON BOARD. Can you imagine hanging off those straps above some bloke who's sitting reading the *Standard* and pointing to your badge smugly . . . I guess that if that didn't work I could whip off my wig, or turban or scarf, and show him my bald head . . .

I am not convinced that I will suit being bald. Some women do. There was that beautiful woman on *Star Trek* (the old TV series) and others. I have no idea if my head is as lumpy as the rest of me? An Indian head masseuse did say once that I had as many bumps as a map of the Himalayas, so I am a little trepidatious. I guess if I do turn out to be that lumpy I can get tattoos on them . . . perhaps a party of skiers or those mountain cows with bells . . . something subtle, of course.

I am going to get there in stages. Stage 1 involves cutting my hair short next week. I rang my hairdresser. He cried. I asked him if he was crying for my hair or for me. It seems to be a bit of both. Once, many years ago, I was going to a premiere and a friend offered to pick me up on a motorbike after I had had my hair done. My hairdresser was incensed that his work of art would be ruined by a helmet and paid for me to have a cab home. Perhaps it is the hair he is attached to.

I know he wants to clone the colour. I have never really known how to describe the colour. I hate 'ginger' and 'red'. I use Titian, Auburn and Strawberry Blonde. My niece calls it 'blorange' which is blonde/orange. I only hope it grows back like that and not the wiry grey pubes I have been warned about. It would be so ironic that after all these years of hating my hair colour it takes the hint and abandons me.

After the bone scan my friend John bought me a book called *Say No to Cancer*. It made me wonder... does anyone say yes? Of course, the book is all about nutrition and lifestyle to avoid cancer. A bit late now. I am tempted to take up chain-smoking and eating red meat for the next five days just to see if I get worse...

This is beyond a joke

5 JUNE 2013

How many more war metaphors can I misappropriate here? There is no doubt that the Eagle Has Landed, built its nest, had eggs, hatched them and sent them to a good local school... I am inexorably bound to this next step. Tomorrow I will be pumped full of toxins. The kind you wouldn't put down your drains to clear out the years of hair and grease in your bathroom pipes. I have had a very surreal day and will write more before I go into the hospital tomorrow morning. Suffice it to say I have had enough of this poor-taste joke... you can tell me now that it has all been a practical joke, ha ha.

The haircut and first day of chemo

6 JUNE 2013

So it started and all things considered it went well. I will update the blog tomorrow as I am a bit woolly-headed but Em and I had a laugh. There were some very funny moments. The funniest was when we checked in on the oncology floor and the receptionist (wearing a burka) said to Em, 'Is it you? It is, isn't it?' and Em replied, 'Yes, it's me but who do you think I am?' Receptionist: 'You were in *The Parent Trap*, weren't you?' to which Em replied, 'That was Natasha Richardson and she's dead.'

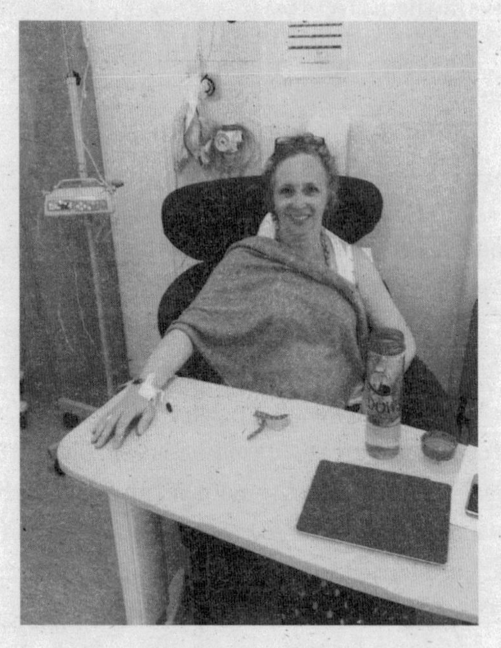

First chemo session – flushing out your veins... I know, right

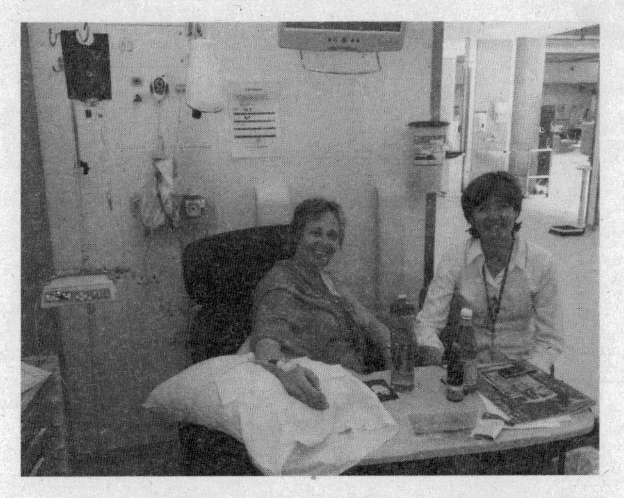

With my cousin Judith who is a nurse at the heart hospital – I am having the last chemical cocktail

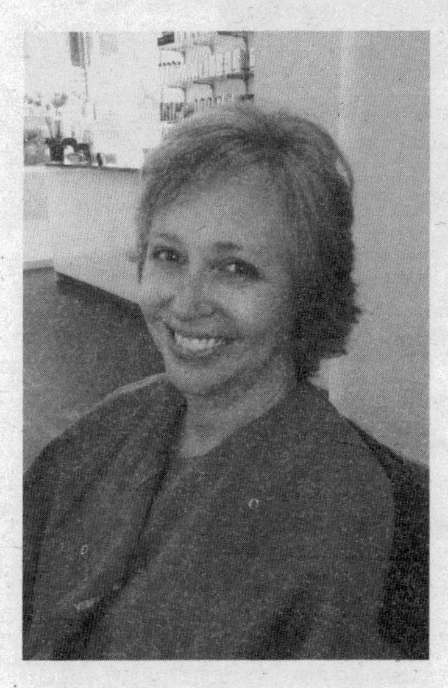

The new haircut –this is my 'disposable haircut' for ten days

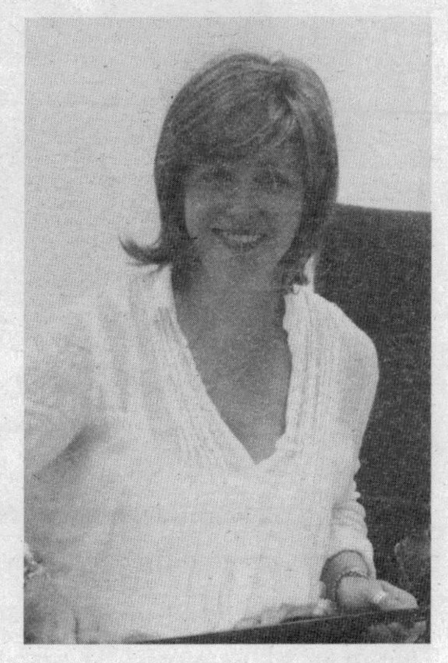

The wig. This NHS wig is called THE CLAIRE – appropriately. Greg thinks I look like a regional TV newsreader

Don't start channelling pond life

7 JUNE 2013

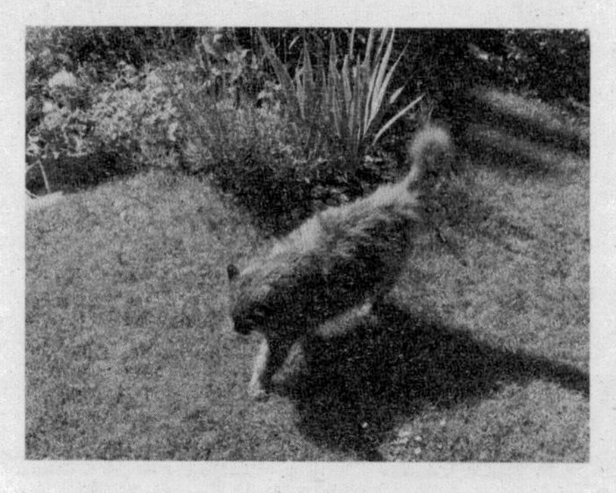

Grablypuss the magnificat – my cat

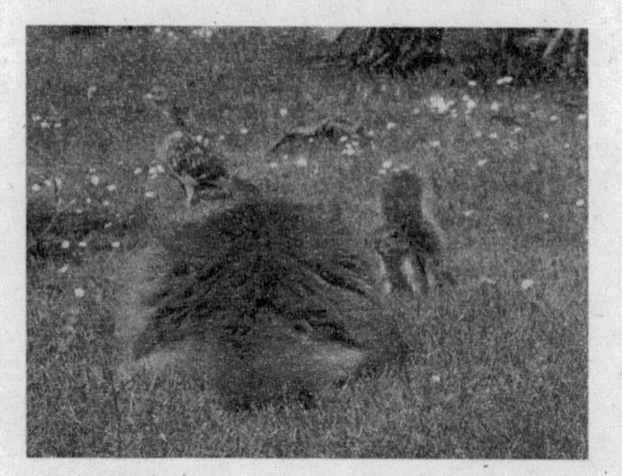

Squirrel chat – soon I shall be channelling all the wildlife here

My lovely friend Peter called me en route from Heathrow to beg me not to start channelling pond life. I told him I only date pond life and have no intention of understanding them. Apparently, he had a neighbour who was one of those people who could suck the joy out of anything. My gran used to refer to them as 'suckers of sour lemons'. Anyway, said lady got diagnosed with terminal cancer, shaved her head and had her chemo. Whilst being treated she discovered that she could channel household pets. And now two years on she has one bestseller book out there and another en route and is a regular on TV breakfast shows. You can look her up – she is called Jackie Weaver.

Can you imagine if I woke up one day during this chemo period able to understand Grablypuss (my cat, for those of you who don't know). I am sure he channels my dead mother because I glimpse him giving me those disapproving looks when I am getting ready to go out. He might well be 'disappointed' in me. It would be like that Mel Gibson film *What Women Want*... it might get noisy on Hampstead Heath with all the dog walkers.

I wanted to also comment about Michael Douglas – I am so intrigued that his throat cancer might have come from oral sex... that would make a lot more sense to me if he were giving men blow jobs but I can't work out the heterosexual danger. I am now worried – how did I get mine? Was it from flaunting my breasts? Rubbing them too much? Giving too much oral sex? Ah no, that was my jaw... blimey, I hope I didn't get cancer in the jaw as well as the fracture.

Back to more toxic news. This whole week has been very odd – getting my hair cut, my teeth cleaned and protected with varnish (I went for a nice teak polish) and then having the pre-chemo assessment which was a little serious and then getting the wig fitted. The staff nurse, who did the pre-chemo stuff, is from Northern Ireland and if I shut my eyes she sounded a bit like the Revd Ian Paisley, although she didn't rant at me. She ran through all the drugs, their side effects and all the arrangements. I think I am now pretty familiar with the swollen ankles, nausea, vomiting, diarrhoea, hair loss, nail blackening, palms and feet itching and general swelling. She also asked me if I was familiar with subcutaneous bolus? No, but I have known a few subhuman bollocks? These are the injections I have to give myself to boost my platelets when I am neutropenic. I asked her if I could travel – not really, as I need to be within an hour of an A & E but I could have the odd day out and I shouldn't travel in planes until I have stopped being neutropenic (no immunity). I asked her if I could do anything fun. Well, you might want sex but it will be uncomfortable and not great, was her reply. Don't worry, I said… if I actually managed to have sex, even when well, it would be announced by the BBC and blessed by the Pope. That warmed her up. I asked about alcohol – 'Bloody hell, yes, if you fancy it with all the shit you're having…' Now this is my kind of medical diagnosis. Phew, so I can still be a pissed sexually attractive Orc.

D-Day arrived and Em and I tripped down to the Cancer Centre and started the five-hour process. The first meeting was with the oncologist who told me that the right breast is fine but lumpy and that the cancer did not respond to some sort of progesterone receptor so I don't have to have Herceptin. She did tell me that my bone scan showed I had fractured a rib a few years ago. I knew it. About three years ago when my friend Gitty was staying he got me stoned (nothing to do with me, of course). I was laughing so hard that I fell into a door jamb. The next morning was agony. When I went to A & E for an X-ray they told me I had just pulled a muscle. Yeah, right. The moral of this story is, if you intend to get stoned and then hysterical stand well clear of walls and furniture.

Thereafter we saw the pharmacist and got all the drugs I have to take home (lots of steroids and anti-nausea tablets). Some of the side effects of the steroids include the condition 'moon face' – can't wait to add that to the list.

Then we went to the chemo floor. My nurse was called Naida and was from the Philippines. She was very nice and after three hours of slow intravenous toxins going into my veins I was rather over the whole experience. Em had done a bit of wandering around and had been recognized by a few people. One Croatian lady came over and talked us through her two bouts of cancer and hysterectomy and said I should lie in bed for six months and pray. It had worked for her. 'Look at me. I am a whale but God loves me,' she said cheerfully when leaving.

Great, add whale to moon face, swollen, etc. etc…

So I feel OK. A bit strange. Last night it felt as though I had jet lag and I was very woolly-headed. I didn't sleep that well but probably due to the steroids (moon face/Arnie) and woke up with metal mouth and slight nausea.

Love, Ms Nuclear 2013

Days 2–3

8 JUNE 2013

I literally bounced out of bed on Day 2, effervescent with energy and all the joys of spring. It was most unexpected. I went to the supermarket, assembled newly acquired garden furniture, started spring-cleaning the shed and contemplated painting it when the rain forced me inside to spring-clean other cupboards. In the evening I tripped up the road for a sumptuous Indian takeaway and some healing red wine. All very normal. I think Greg was very relieved as he had been away this last week and probably was expecting the worst. I put it down to all the steroids I have had both intravenously and also in pill form.

Several friends have asked me to pop over and do spring-cleaning at their houses and I did even consider it. Strike whilst the iron is hot and all that…

Day 3 has not been quite so energetic, but I am still functioning reasonably well and have managed to be up and about, do some gardening and read a bit. Again, not what I was expecting but don't get me wrong, I am thrilled.

I have to take my temperature twice a day. So far it has been around the 33.1 to 34.1 mark, very low. I suspect that the final blue chemo was antifreeze. If my temperature rises above 38 (normal is 37.5ish) I have to go to hospital, but being cold-blooded doesn't seem to be a problem. Perhaps I am turning amphibian like in *X-Men*. I hope I do get a superpower after all of this. I am not sure I want to channel animals or even develop cold blood but something extra would be nice. Right now I would settle for reading without my glasses.

I am going to update this page of the blog every few days. I don't want to bombard you with emails unless I have something interesting to say, like first hair loss.

Thanks for all your great comments and love. x

Day 4

9 JUNE 2013

I suspect they injected me with cleaning fluid. I have been on a spring-cleaning hype and cannot get over how well I am feeling so far – very busy and fizzy with all the steroids. My temperature is still very low, around 33… I am a little like the Duracell Bunny in that I am slowly running out of juice and have started a little slower today. The steroids are finished so maybe the adrenaline push is over and I am about to let the toxins into my body.

However, despite the slowing down I have done a Tesco shop and been to a garden centre so I can plant up some veg. I am becoming much more interested in the subject of food and healing – I don't think my body will ever be a temple but it might stop being a roadside truck stop.

xxx

Days 6–8

13 JUNE 2013

I am thrilled to report that I am actually still doing pretty well. I suspect that the chemo is mixed with cleaning fluid (as well as antifreeze) as I am still on a major cleaning kick. I have even treated myself to new pillows and new bedding in anticipation of spending more time in bed. I realized that I was still using pillows on my bed from my university days – that can't be good.

Today (Day 8) I have had to be given a subcutaneous bolus – an injection into the fleshy part of my tummy. Luckily there was lots of flesh to choose from. I am debating whether to post the photo of it (the injection being given, not the fleshy bits) but there is such a wide geographical area of upper thigh and abdomen on display it would put anyone off their tea. The injection is to stimulate the white platelets. It makes your bones ache but is not too bad. Em, my sister-in-law, came over to give it to me... I must admit she was very enthusiastic at the thought of sticking me with a needle. Another friend suggested I should get a nurse to do it but Em has played an award-winning cancer patient in *Wit* so she's virtually medically trained.

Strangely, apart from feeling a little fluey and having a low temperature still, I am not really experiencing any symptoms. However, I had not expected to feel anything when my hair falls out (apart from the obvious emotional impact) but it does hurt. You know that feeling when you part your hair differently or sleep awkwardly and the roots ache... well, that's what my whole head feels like. Apparently, the roots are getting ready to jump ship and are dying. So far there haven't been handfuls of hair but the process is clearly starting. I may well keep it and mix with the cat fur to create small creatures or stuff cushions. Clare Bear Hair Inc. as someone suggested.

I am still debating about more fun wigs – Sanjeev suggested a seventies' Afro so I could look blaxploitation kick-ass – in my case more whiteploitation. I think it's an excellent idea. An old friend from school thinks I should go for *Hit Girl from Kick-Ass*. These are all definite possibilities. Mark, who is staying with me, told me not to discount Maggie Thatcher style. Not sure I can pull that off at my young age, although she was probably this age when she was styled as Maggie.

Off to the hospital tomorrow for blood tests. Almost halfway through first chemo bout. I worked out the chemo period is 126 days in total (if all goes according to plan) and I am on Day 8 – so far so good. If I really don't start developing major recognizable symptoms soon people are going to doubt whether I really do have cancer.

Bring on the bald. xxx

Wet dreams and nipple piercing

15 JUNE 2013

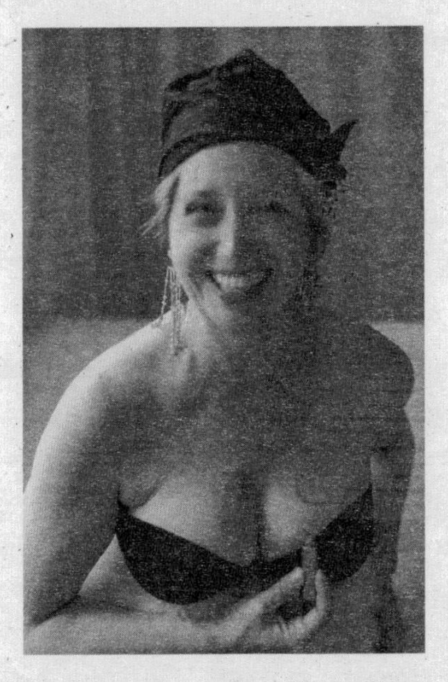

I think this one says it all. I will upload a whole lot of fabulous pics that Richard took yesterday. And there will be a competition for best caption

A few years ago a wet dream meant titillation and excitement and that in theory I was still sexually active. Now a wet dream is just exactly that... WET. Yuck, cold clammy and soaked through. Chemo does propel you into perimenopause and then menopause. So far only the night sweats which are really unpleasant. Thank goodness I sleep alone (apart from the cat).

Philly reckons that the cat is a husband/boyfriend from a former life as ever since he appeared in mine (fourteen and a half years ago) it has been nigh on impossible for me to have sex. At first it was funny. When he was a kitten I audaciously walked into a very trendy bar in Westbourne Grove and basically acted like a cougar and picked up a young man who literally grabbed his satchel in haste to follow me home. He was not, I should add, underage but had just graduated from uni (making him around twenty-one and I was definitely the other side of thirty) and was working as a scientist in a petroleum company and he had to carry this enormous adrenaline syringe with him at all times – it was like the one in *Pulp Fiction*. Basically, if there was a gas leak he had to be stabbed through the heart with it. Crikey.

Emboldened by my trampish behaviour I took him home and showed him a good time – in fact, it was more like an interactive lesson in women. Young men really don't need any sleep and are very eager to please. (Apologies to my family here who may be reading this in disgust.) In the midst of Lesson 1 the cat, who was really little, sat beside the bed and every time I made any kind of noise, he miaowed. The young man asked me in between bouts if it was me making the strange noise . . . I told him that's how cougars get their name. They miaow during sex.

Since then Grablypuss has made appearances during sex which have included jumping on one bloke's back, insisting on sitting on my head purring (nothing like that to put off a Romeo), and squeezing in between us to lie protectively on my tummy. Some of you out there are puzzled as to why I didn't shut him out – I lived in a house with no door handles so the cat had no difficulty opening doors. But why didn't I put him in the garden? It's worse having him sit at the window by the bed crying and pawing the window, believe me. That also puts a chap off his game.

The other night I woke to find the cat with a protective paw laid over my diseased breast. I do think Philly might be right.

And now to nipple piercing – I have to go into the hospital to have titanium clips put onto the tumour so that the doctors can monitor whether the tumour shrinks in chemo. So I will have expensive internal nipple piercing. Imagine explaining that at Heathrow security.

Richard came round last night to take more photos and I am modelling a range of chemo headgear – the best comments left by you guys will garner a prize – maybe a lock of my hair or a small creature knitted from a combo of my hair and Grably's fur. Or perhaps just a bottle of wine.

Let me know your thoughts.

Clare x

Side effects at last…

16 JUNE 2013

Just when you all thought that I was escaping very lightly, I have developed two side effects. The first is small but unbelievably painful (I am a wuss). I have two mouth ulcers either side of the back of my mouth at gum level. I try to cover them with Bonjela but the bloody thing just slips down my throat and it tastes awful. The only positive side to mouth ulcers is that I really can't eat much. A good thing as along with the cleaning fluid and antifreeze they injected me with, the chemo made me hungry. That's not supposed to happen – I am supposed to emerge from this experience stick thin and healthy. At this rate I will turn into a whale.

The other side effect is very bizarre and painful. I had my second injection for stimulating the bone marrow to produce more white blood cells to help me fight infection whilst I am neutropenic (no immunity) and mid-chemo. The side effect of this was to make every bone not just ache but sing out in pain. I literally lay down and could feel my whole skeleton from the skull, through each vertebra of my spine, each rib and in particular the pelvis and how the legs fitted there. It felt as though my bones were trying to escape my body. It was the weirdest feeling and definitely the worst side effect so far.

I also couldn't bend or make sudden movements, like turning. I started to walk like a zombie (more *Shaun of the Dead* than *World War Z*), which was actually very funny. For the next cycle I might loan myself out to Paramount for their marketing campaign for *World War Z*. I even groaned once or twice in a way that George A. Romero would have approved of... I see a moneymaking opportunity opening up. Perhaps I won't have to knit my own hair.

Steph reminded me that once when I had flu I complained that my hair ached. He said no one has ever described their hair as aching. Weirdly, he also doesn't get teeth itch... is it just me? I do have times when my teeth itch. Anyway, this is apropos of my scalp still aching but so far I still have a healthy head of hair. A disappointment, I know.

Off to hospital tomorrow for the internal nipple piercing.

Clare x

Anything but ginger

18 JUNE 2013

I have been studiously avoiding any books with personal accounts of cancer. Having said that, though, I do trawl through their indexes looking for side effects and seeing if they tally with what I've come to expect. They do. But several people, including that spiffing BBC Radio parliamentary correspondent, recommended *Love for Now* by the poet Anthony Wilson. He was diagnosed with non-Hodgkins lymphoma and decided to write about his chemo experience. When he was being told that his hair might grow back a different colour he said, and I quote, 'Please, God, not ginger.'

Today whilst waiting for my meds at the Cancer Centre I overheard a nurse briefing a chap about what to expect from the side effects of the chemo. She ran through the familiar list and when she got to the hair bit and explained his hair might come back curly and a different colour he too exclaimed, 'Anything but ginger.' Hmm. We 'redheads', flame-haired, Titian locks, auburn, blorange people, could really take offence. We are already stigmatized by everyone knowing that it is a recessive gene that produces strawberry-blonde hair. Isn't that enough? I was the only little girl in my primary school with this colour hair and I was bullied for it all the way through school.

There was only one time in my life when I thought it was a major advantage. I was about eight and Greg was seven and we were due to go on holiday to Tunisia, but Greg got mumps and there was a revolution anyway. So instead the parents did something completely out of character for them. They booked a beach holiday to a place near Lisbon in Portugal. Most of our holidays were spent visiting churches, cathedrals, art galleries, stately homes, chateaux and famous buildings (both my parents were architects) and if we were very good we could have half a day or even a full one on a beach or in a park. To get ice creams we had to not spill on tablecloths at restaurants. Suddenly I see my parents' whole parenting rationale – bribery.

Anyway, this was a totally different holiday: we had to visit two cathedrals and a castle but basically it was more beach than culture. But everywhere I went little old ladies dressed in their black outfits with their heads covered in mantillas, would come up to me, touch my head and make the sign of the cross. I was in. I was the Madonna.

Years later, when I became a tour guide (you see, all that traipsing around places of interest paid off), I met a Portuguese guide and asked him if I was the Madonna and should I move to Portugal to marry their king or whatever they had available... He laughed. It was more than just a laugh – it looked genuinely painful when he was doubled up going purple in the face. Madonna? No.

Apparently, when the Vikings were raiding Europe in the eighth century they landed in Portugal and did their mandatory raping and pillaging and every so often there's a genetic memory of the shame of succumbing to the Vikings and a child is born with red hair. In effect, the women are crossing themselves to say, 'Thank God she's not mine.'

Hmmm. I still have my hair and it is still blorange.

Anthony Wilson did spend quite a lot of his book getting on his high horse about the phrase 'battling' with cancer. He particularly resented journalists and presenters describing someone as 'having lost the fight with cancer'. As he says, it's not a battle or a fight.

I think I agree in part with him. I am certainly not at war with my tumour. I am more of a voyeur in the fight between chemicals and multi-divisional bad cells. In fact, I am sort of the battlefield and rather passive in the whole process. My only role is to provide a venue.

I did go to the hospital today and had the internal nipple piercing done. I then had three mammograms. Ouch, ouch, ouch. I asked if there was a similar machine for men's testicles. No. They only use ultrasound on men because they are less complex (the testicles compared to the breast). I still think it's a conspiracy.

The very exciting news is that I am on Day 14 (out of 126) and my tumour has shrunk from 3.5 centimetres to 3.4 centimetres. If I could do the maths I would work out how long it would take to shrink completely, etc. etc., but for now I am just glad it is shrinking. Here is a picture of several things that are 3.5 centimetres long – a matchbox, a strand of All Bran (odd choice, I know), a dishwasher tablet. In fact, the dishwasher tablet is a useful comparison as the tumour is almost as thick as the tablet as well.

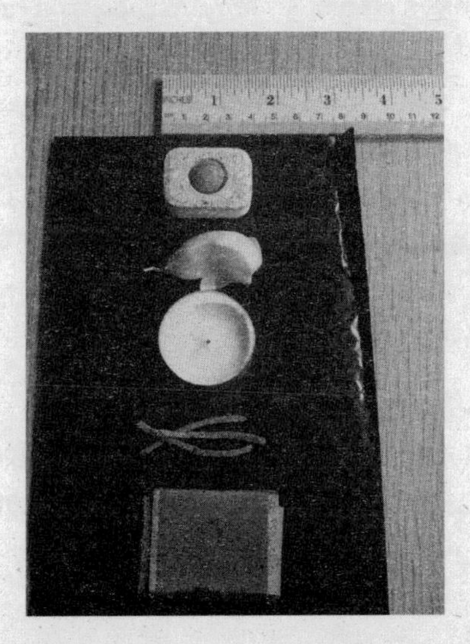

I also got some novocaine for my mouth ulcers . . . yippee. I will now be able to take solid foods again.

The flame/Titian/auburn/blorange Clare x

Bald: the final frontier

20 JUNE 2013

These are the voyages of the Starship *Clarewise* to baldly go seeking out . . .

Enough *Star Trek.* It's finally happening. I have deciduous hair, coming out in handfuls, and I expect that I will be 'bald as a coot' (must look up the origin of that saying) by early next week.

Weirdly, this does feel like the final frontier. Once this has happened there's no going back and pretending it's not real. Don't worry, I am not maudlin. My Marilyn Monroe wig arrived today – I think it is made of AstroTurf but will be fun for at least one wear.

As I said, I had been studiously avoiding books on cancer but since my insomnia, I have taken to dipping in and out of recipe books and the odd 'self-help' ones given to me. One called *Anticancer: A new way of life* is written by a neuroscientist and he looks at psychological connections. There is a lot of debate here in the UK about the link between breast cancer and stress. It seems that the oncologists are not sure it can be proven but the psychologists feel that there is an empirical link.

I don't know about psychologists and science. When I was very little (three or four) I had a friend called Wendy who lived next door. Her parents were behavioural psychologists at the university. They were testing obedience versus natural instinct. One day they told Wendy to throw a milk bottle at the telly – clearly they wanted to see if she would do as they asked or refuse because it would kill the telly. Needless to say she did it and they had a broken telly. I wanted to do the same experiment at home but for some reason my parents were less keen. So much for my psychological development.

In the past I have tried meditation and mindfulness. My friend Emma and I did a short one-day course. I was still working at the studio and fair to say I was somewhat stressed and tired – so when we were told to relax and get comfortable, I fell asleep. She says I snored but I know that was someone else . . . a lady never snores.

I have a different kind of stress right now and I think it could be time to learn meditation properly. My stepfather Imre (a Hungarian) had a heart condition and practised yoga and meditation. One day when I was visiting with a boyfriend (I was at Cambridge so it was aeons ago, before Grably and also when I still knew some straight men), the cat from next door came in and jumped on my lap. Imre turned to Jamie and said very authoritatively, 'Stroking pussy reduces blood pressure.'

So now you know . . . Grablypuss, come here.

Handfuls of hair

24 JUNE 2013

I woke up this morning and found what looked like a rodent but turned out to be a large fistful of hair. The shower took out about half my head of hair. I just hope I don't get a comb over . . . but either way everyone said, Day 18, your hair goes. And guess what? It's Day 18 and I never ever thought I would be predictable . . . more later.

Bald as a coot

25 JUNE 2013

Shaving my head – with a little help from my family.

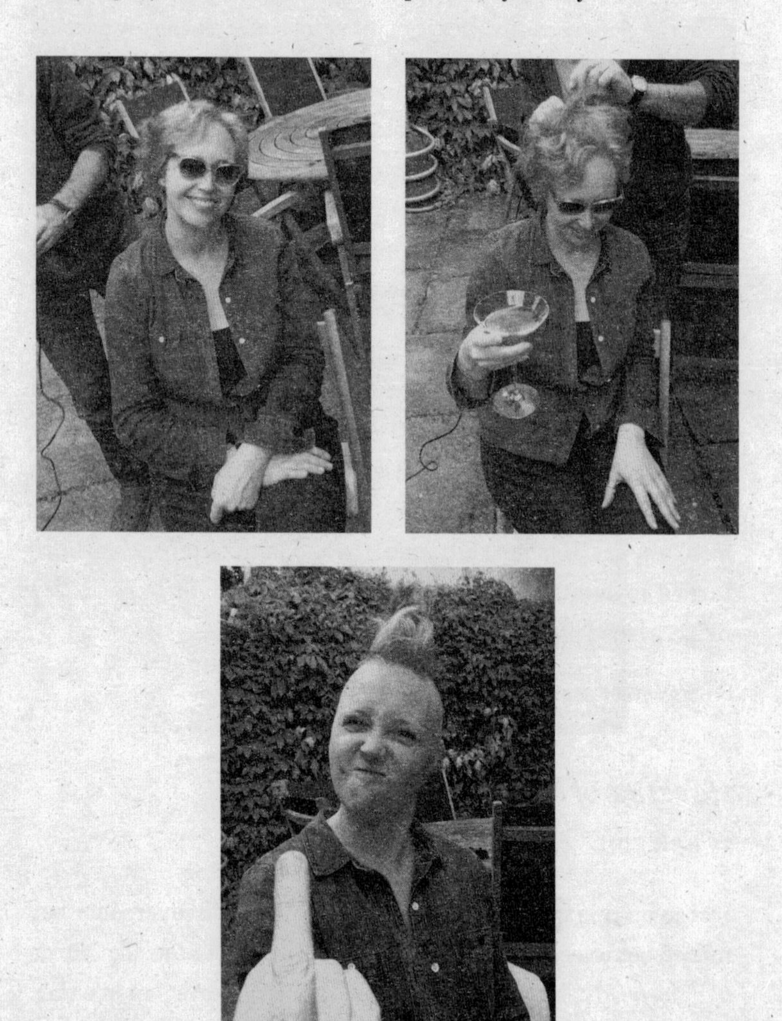

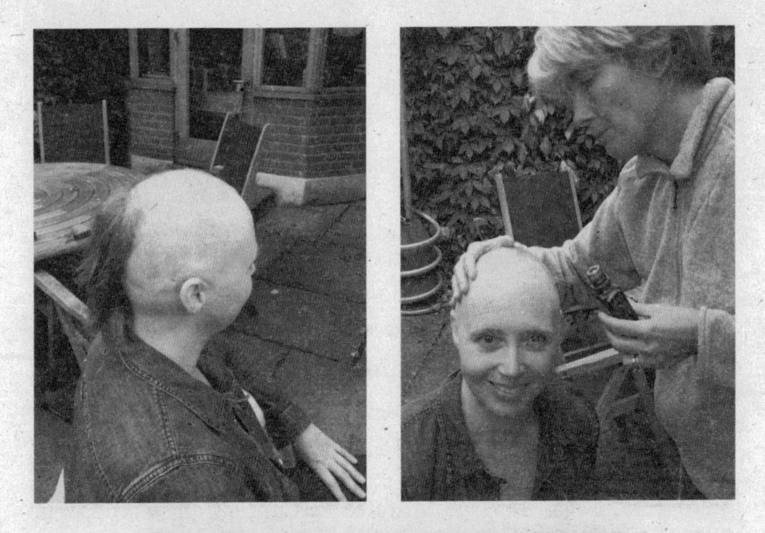

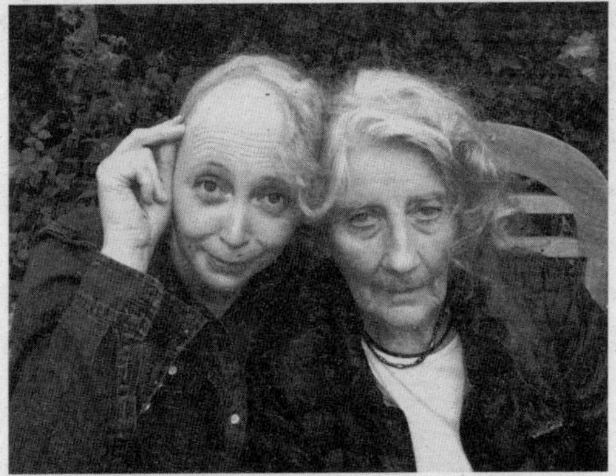

The gorgeous older woman is Phyllida Law, the actress and very successful author. Her hair is down to her waist so I may be borrowing some. Greg was the hairdresser, Em the stylist and Gaia, my niece, the photographer. I suspect they may have had some fun at my expense – a Mohawk, a Hare Krishna limp ponytail????

My head feels very light and cold. Last night I slept in a bed cap. I am turning into a Dickensian character. Theoretically, I am going on the town tonight. I feel a little nervous about being seen in public. Odd really, after exposing myself on this blog.

Chemo Round 2

26 JUNE 2013

Tomorrow I am back in the hospital for Round 2 of complete poisoning. The difference this time is that I know what to expect from the actual day of being given chemo and now I look like an egg with a body... I am worried that I do have a bit of a cone-head.

I think I will wear Gloria Swanson to the Cancer Centre to cheer up my nurses and oncologist and the other patients. Let them think I am eccentric rather than just headwear-challenged.

I will report back... expect side effects this time as chemo is cumulative. In fact, I am told that it takes almost two years for the cytoxic drugs (my current FEC chemo) to leave your body. In the same Internet search I also discovered that it takes two weeks for marijuana to leave your system and four for cocaine. Not that I am checking or anything...

I also learned that 'bald as a coot' dates back to the fifteenth century. Those poor birds – they just don't get a break, do they?

Some lovely ex-colleagues have sent me DVDs to cheer me up – the first one out of the envelope was *Schindler's List* – not sure that is cheering, but a great film.

First night out with Gloria Swanson turban

28 JUNE 2013

For the first time I hit the town. A meeting at BAFTA, where everyone was very nice about the turban (the one with the large Swarovski brooch). Then a drink at the Groucho, with my lovely friend, and fab lawyer, Charles. As we were walking to dinner, a chap was hit by a car and fell head first onto the pavement in front of us. Luckily I have been watching a lot of *House* and saw his head injury. I applied pressure, had him sit down, talk to me about his life, and Charles phoned for an ambulance.

The lesson is that I shouldn't leave the 'hood apart from chemo.

Slight delay in normal transmission

30 JUNE 2013

Apologies to everyone looking for a post-chemo Round 2 update, but this one has flattened me and I haven't even had the energy to blog. I haven't been wrapped around the loo, but I have been nauseous and wiped out. Walking to the kitchen and back to bed has felt like a marathon. I will update blog tomorrow, which, hopefully, will be a better day.

The bald and the beautiful

2 JULY 2013

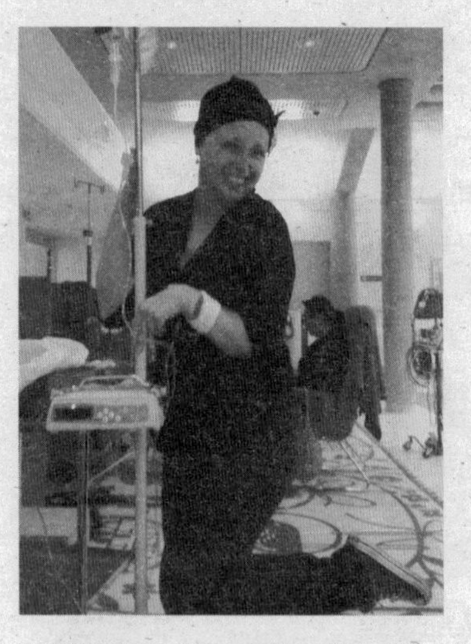

Gloria Swanson does chemo

Normal service is resumed. Apologies for the crippling lethargy aka chemo fatigue that has prevented me from updating the blog and in fact from doing anything now for six days. But that's a thing of the past and today I am firing on at least one cylinder.

Last Thursday I was nuked for the second time. Before each chemo session your blood has to be analysed – first for haemoglobin and then for renal and liver functions. Ideally, blood work should be done the day before, but like every test in my life I left it to the last moment. I will never learn, and assumed that I could blag the four-hour blood delay by being chirpy, but it turns out that there is a good reason for the four hours. That's how long it takes.

I found myself on the Tube in rush hour. Never a pleasant experience, and even less so when you are going into hospital. I decided to pull the 'poor me, I have cancer' gag and get a seat. My first (and actually only) victim was a nicely dressed twenty-something bloke en route to the City. I first tried to just look sick (no dice), I even took a puff of my inhaler (he didn't flinch or look up from his Game Boy). Then I went in for the kill.

'I'd like to sit down, please, or would you rather I show you my bald head?' He very hastily vacated both the seat and the Tube car. Perhaps he thought I was a cross butch woman – or maybe he feared cancer was catching. I felt a small amount of smugness and then deflated. Although I have wanted to be treated equally, I do still want some doors opened for me and a seat on a crowded train. Am I a hypocrite? Yes, no, possibly. I am definitely indecisive. My only decision is to discuss a badge with London Transport, as mentioned before like the 'Baby on Board' one, only for tumours.

I do still stand for someone older than me, male or female, or mums with infants, etc. Sometimes I have been the only woman on a Tube car and have still been the one to stand up. I feel very old and bitter all of a sudden about manners.

Anyway, the bald bitter bitch made it to the department of phlebotomy – isn't that a great name? It is apparently from the Greek. Most of the staff are very friendly Albanians. That's where they draw the blood and do some analysis and the rest is sent to haematology. I am beginning to feel resentful at all the blood that's being taken from me. Also, rather bizarrely, I don't know my blood group and will have to remember to ask next time I am with the vampires. I make them laugh, as before any nurse or doctor can stick a needle into you, they have to ask you your name and your date of birth. I always give my birth date and then tell them I am thinking about going younger. The female nurses think I could easily get away with five years and the males with ten. Not sure what that says about the sexes, but perhaps I can get a research grant to investigate it...

Before being poisoned you have to be seen by the oncology team and the pharmacist. I met the latest member of my team and the one in whose name a lot of the tests have been carried out. She is based partly at the Cancer Centre and partly at the Royal Free. She loved the Gloria Swanson turban, but has given me a challenge – for me to come as a different film star to each chemo session. I have the Marilyn wig, I am getting a Rasta one (not sure if there's a film star in that, but I could act out *Cool Runnings*), so now we just have to think of rocking starlets for the next four sessions.

Since my blood work wasn't done, we had to wait for hours. So long, that I was begging my nurse to give me chemo. I never thought I would be pleading for poison. The second round of drugs was the same as the first – this heady cocktail called FEC. My fabulous and brilliant and brave friend Philippa came to the chemo with me. She had virtually the same cancer eighteen months ago, but was treated in a much more medieval and draconian fashion at a hospital that is not spanking new and light and airy. Her chemo experience could not be more different than mine. She quite rightly pointed out that all the chemo floor needs is some mood lighting and a bar and it could be a West London hotel. I think I will mention that on the feedback form – they could also do with some of that chillax music from the Buddha Bar.

That evening my niece, Gaia, and nephew, Tindy, were coming to dinner. Tindy has been living in Cairo for the last six months. He has been doing something amazing and inspiring: helping refugees there by setting up a centre where they can get legal advice, meet others in similar positions, do poetry evenings or express themselves creatively. He got out of Cairo just before the anniversary of Morsi's coming to power, which as expected has been violent. As I write I am assuming that by tomorrow the army will be in power again there.

Anyway, he was very happy to be home. He was particularly happy to see women's heads and bodies and not just their ankles peeking out from a burka. I guess some things don't change then.

By the next day and for the five days after I have felt as though someone picked me up and slammed me against a wall and then ran me over with a steamroller and unplugged my power source. Walking from my bed to the kitchen has felt like the ascent on Everest and I have had to stop at Base Camp (sofa) in both directions. Luckily I haven't felt too nauseous, but just literally I stopped like the bunnies that aren't powered by Duracell. This is a well-recognized side effect and it's called fatigue. No shit, Sherlock.

The steroids have not made me want to clean or bounce around but they are inflating me like a rotund Humpty Dumpty. Surely not eating for five days shouldn't make you gain weight. But that's the beauty of cancer. You cannot eat, and throw up your guts, but you still put on the pounds. Welcome to my own inner Circle of Hell.

The good news is that I am on Day 27 of 126 days, so we are already into double digits.

Hair today…gone tomorrow

5 JULY 2013

I thought I would look up some of the words I have been bandying about. (For those of you under sixteen, I used a book called an *Encyclopedia* – it is an antique form of Wikipedia and you can use it without needing WiFi. It may yet catch on.)

ALOPECIA – from the Ancient Greek for fox – specifically fox mange. Apparently a fox sheds its coat twice a year. I feel it is yet another aspersion about being ginger dressed up as an obscure fact about a fox.

BALD – this is an old English word(e) '*balde*' which means white or pale. It is a bastardization of a Celtic word used to describe piebald horses.

FATIGUE – first identified in the 1660s as 'that which causes weariness' from the French for tired '*fatigué*' and the Latin '*fatigare*' which means to break down. '*Fati-agos*' means driven to the point of breakdown or weariness from exertion. Before cancer I honestly thought that I had been fatigued before – heavy jet lag, all-nighters at university are NOTHING compared to chemo fatigue. It is quite literally as though the power has been switched off.

BREAST – from a Gothic word '*Brusts*' which means swelling or to sprout.

MASTECTOMY – Greek word for breast is '*mastos*'. Hence an Amazonian warrior is so called not because of where they came from but because they reputedly burnt off their left breasts so that they could be better archers. '*A*' means 'without' and '*mastos*' is breast.

CHEMO BRAIN – two days ago I called the shed a fridge and am on the whole very forgetful and sometimes peter out in the middle of a sentence. I seem to be doing a lot of charades to get my point across. It must be endlessly entertaining for my companions.

The Good, the Bald and the Ugly

7 JULY 2013

Richard came over and took some more pictures – we decided on one glam shot and then three bald film stars. Got to have some fun with the bald head.

Thanks to Gaia and Greg for the styling and prosthetics and Richard for the photography and Fi, Esther, Grant and Gitty for laughing.

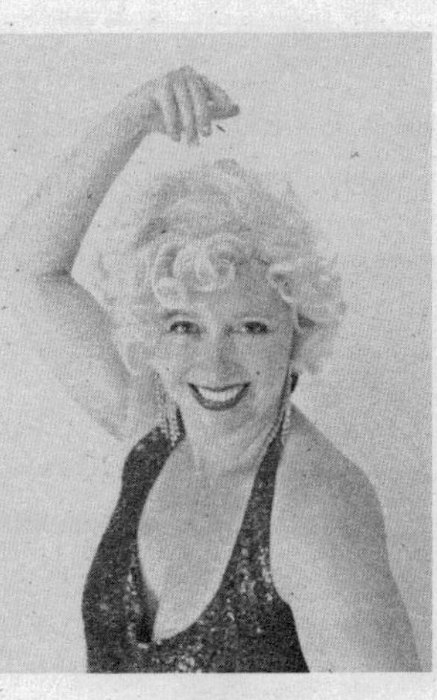

Clarelyn

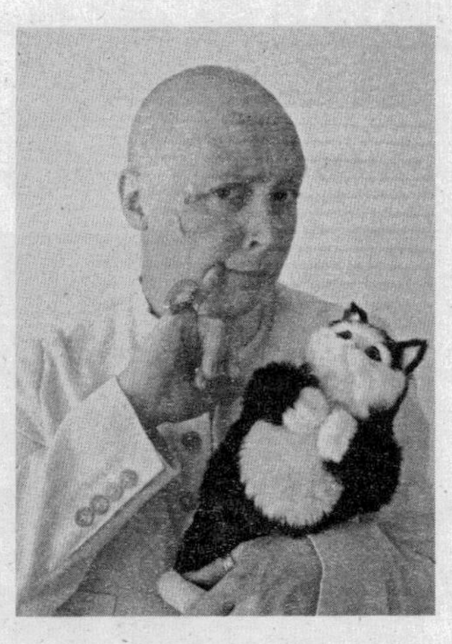

Dr Weevil

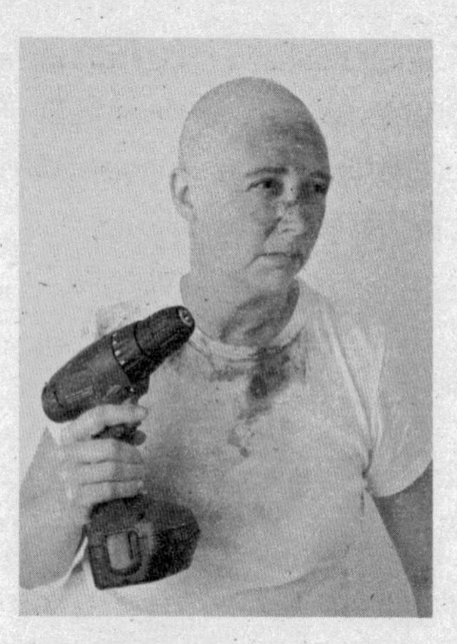

DIY-Hard Another Day

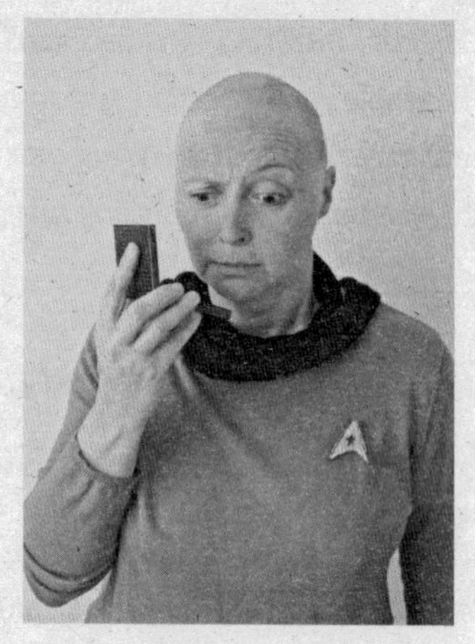

Picard to Bridge

Talking of Facebook . . .

9 JULY 2013

I have been amazed at the response to my blog both from people I know (you kind of have to say nice things) and from strangers.

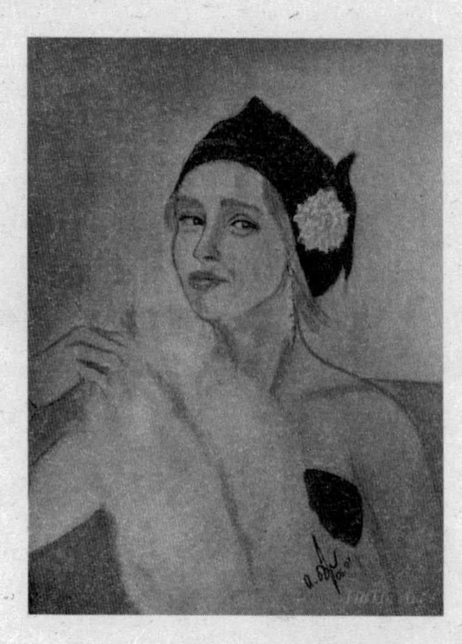

This portrait is a gift from Tina who is from Tbilisi in Georgia and is an artist who came across my blog through Facebook. I can't even find myself on Facebook so I am in awe of her talents.

Talking of Facebook: yesterday I learned a new Facebook-related word from my niece – she had left her computer open on her FB page and a friend had posted something rude. Apparently her page had been FRAPED – I can only assume this means Facebook-raped. I don't know whether to be more shocked about the posting or the fraping word.

Next chemo is on Thursday – hopefully. I am still in hypothermia – my body temperature finally reached a high of 36 (normal is around 39) and for the last seven weeks I have been hovering around 33. It had reached 36 because I seem to have caught some kind of chill. I think when I came out of neutropenia I assumed I could be normal so we went out at night to a picnic concert in Kew Gardens with Howard Jones supporting the Human League – yes, the eighties are back with a vengeance and there is even an eighties fashion exhibition at the V&A. It was fantastic, but late, and there was a cold wind blowing. Phil Oakey has gone even balder than me. I didn't realize that the Human League have sold over 20 million records and have even released new tracks. Sadly for them, no one is interested in their new material. I was surprised how many tracks I knew and the memories of school discos and embarrassing crushes, fumbled kisses, etc., that the music evoked. What was particularly funny was all the bad 'Dad dancing' and kids lying around on Game Boys asking if they could go home to bed now at 10 p.m.

Rock chick meets chemo chick

12 JULY 2013

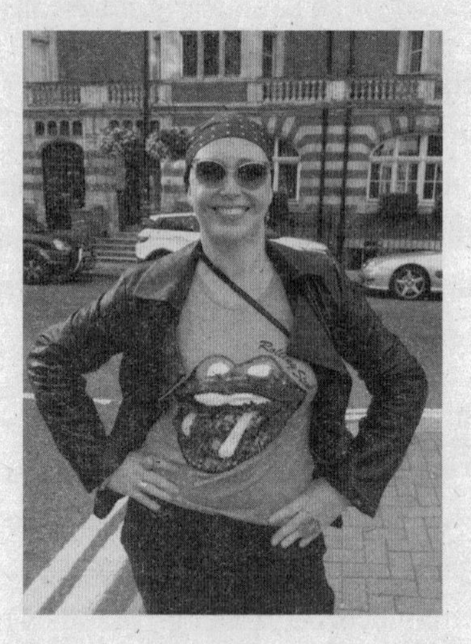

I have been feeling really so much better since last week. I am sure that has to do with the start of summer – HURRAH – which coincided with the saintly Esther coming from Australia to look after me until September. I now have my own personal valet, houseboy, driver and chef. It's going to be hard to let her go home. She has given me very strict instructions I am allowed to pootle and potter (there is a subtle difference, I promise) and procrastinate but not allowed to do anything that involves me moving too much. I could really milk this.

We (family) had been promised tickets to see the Rolling Stones in Hyde Park, but when the organizers found out that Em wasn't able to be there, our tickets were rescinded. I was a little upset as that meant that twice I had been prevented from seeing the Stones live in concert – in 1982 they played Roundhay Park in Leeds and I was doing my O levels and so my parents wouldn't let me go.

Anyway, my amazing and fabulous brother managed to track down Marlon Richards, son of Keith, who organized for us to apply for tickets. Greg paid an arm and a leg for them – which might hold back his career a bit – but refused to allow me to pay him back even with a pound of flesh to make up for the loss of limbs.

It was a fabulous evening. The park had been open since noon and a lot of very sunburnt, drunk people had waited until 8.30 p.m. to hear the Stones. There were lots of other bands far too trendy and up-to-date for me to know. None of them has appeared on Radio 4. The Stones are on a fiftieth-anniversary tour and the Hyde Park gigs are a repeat of their 1969 concert, which was a few days after Brian Jones died and was free. This time 65,000 people inside the walled-off area paid to see them, and another 5,000 sat outside and heard it for free. There were also some people as old as the band, who rocked on down and smoked spliffs and generally seemed to think it was still 1969.

Mick and 'the boys' put me to shame – for two hours they played and moved around like sprightly young things. Mick strutted and preened and jumped and sang and played the mouth organ and the guitar as though he were someone a quarter his age. He is seventy, Charlie Watts is seventy-two (he looked as though he had forgotten his teeth but apart from that drummed solidly for two hours). The amazing medical anomaly is the death-defying survivor Keith Richards. Surely being an addict for forty-five years should have taken more of a toll on him. He looked just as ravaged – but with his bandana and eye make-up and sallow skin, the only thing that gave him away as a septuagenarian were his ears. They really do keep growing all your life. I wonder with my chemo, which is killing off parts of me still growing, whether my ears stop for this period?

They were bloody marvellous. I pulled the chemo-cancer-chick card to get into our area without fighting through the crowds and we had a fabulous time.

What was a real reminder of times past was that all the band (bar Mick) smoked on stage and casually flicked their cigarettes for minions to extinguish. They must be the last people on the planet allowed to smoke and still be role models.

Apparently Mick does hours of yoga and Pilates every day and runs eight miles to de-stress. All this at seventy. I think I might follow the Jagger regime (without the running and years of drug abuse).

Rock (chemo) chick x

Good things about cancer

15 JULY 2013

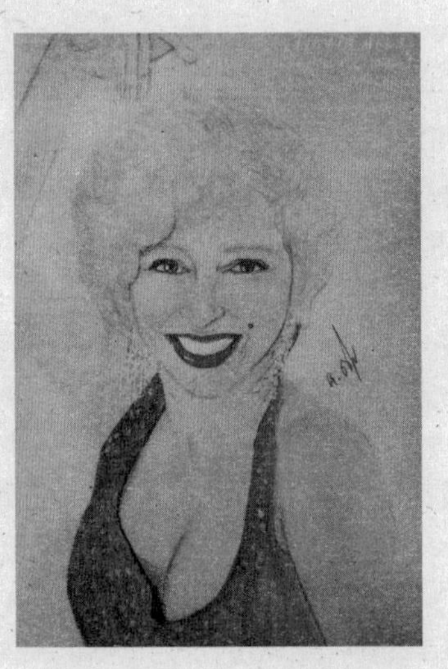

Tina from Georgia did another portrait

There are really some wonderful things about having cancer (not that I would ever actively go out and recommend you try for cancer…) and I have had some fantastic experiences.

No. 1 Friends – I am very lucky in that so many friends are in touch constantly and sending me cards, emails and calling. I have even got back in touch with loved and missed friends scattered all over the world. I am very lucky that Esther has come all the way from Australia to look after me for two months. Everyone has been fantastic – as have my family, of course. I have never felt alone or upset. There are so many people sending me good wishes.

I have had a few little wobbles – the day my hair fell out in handfuls was really the only time I had a little cry. I haven't gone through the five stages of grief the doctors etc. tell you to expect. I may well still be in Stage 1 – denial. I am not angry or bitter (the 'why me?' stage) and I am not depressed and I am not sure that I am accepting the cancer or just going with the flow. The whole process is fascinating – from the twice-daily temperature check (I am still hypothermic) to changes in taste in my mouth, learning new things about my body and my condition.

No. 2 Making new friends – like Tina who very sweetly has done another portrait of me as Marilyn. I am very flattered by her attention.

I have also made wonderful friends at the hospital – phenomenally dedicated staff, nurses and also volunteers. Yesterday I did a session at the Macmillan Centre which is sponsored by a charity called Look Good, Feel Better – please look them up at www.lgfb.co.uk. The UK beauty and health care industry puts together goody bags and holds a pampering class for every woman with cancer all over the country. They provide make-up artists to help women feel better about using cosmetics when they are sick, have no hair, etc. It was a wonderful afternoon – I was with six women of all ages and types. There was a very young and very sick girl and even she managed to feel a bit better after our session. I am going to try and do something for this organization and also for Macmillan – who are quite frankly brilliant. I will hold Macmillan's The World's Biggest Coffee Morning event which is in September and force neighbours and friends to buy cupcakes and maybe even get my niece to do it at school. I really can't say enough about this organization and the people who work for it.

No. 3 Save on shampoo – yes, I have finally come round to realizing that being bald in this hot weather is actually a blessing. I am also always tempted by '3 for the price of 2' hair offers and trying new shampoos so I am probably saving myself a tidy sum by not indulging. Yesterday I took the Tube to the hospital – OMG in temperatures of over 30 degrees centigrade we were squashed in like cattle and I found myself nestling under a very smelly armpit. On my return journey I demanded a seat from a chap sitting in that seat that says, 'Please give up for someone in need.' In France it used to say 'mutilated in the war', which sounds much more dramatic. I whipped off my hat to show that I was mutilated and in need of the seat. He was very grumpy. I suspect it was the heat.

No. 4 Having the opportunity to make changes in your life and lifestyle; I am not proselytizing about a pure life – I will never be that good – but I do have a chance to make some changes, especially vis-à-vis stress levels and diet and health. I am hoping that I will be better about what I eat and drink. I haven't really managed to give up alcohol in my good weeks as I have convinced myself that a daily glass (or two/three) of red wine is good for my iron levels. Philly has been brilliant about giving up all dairy and red meat and alcohol. If I can get within a gnat's crotchet of her diet I will be doing very well.

As I think I have mentioned before, bizarrely chemo does make you hungry. Not the first week, which is pretty much overtaken by nausea and cravings for ginger and salt and spicy foods. But the week of neutropenia and also the third good week I could basically just graze all day like a fat dairy cow.

No.5 Lolling around – it's very nice to loll and not feel guilty. I don't have the brain for reading much but enjoy just hanging.

No. 6 Catching up on TV series I have missed. Colleen gave me *Friday Night Lights* Series 3 and I am saving that for next chemo bed week. I got to Series 4 of *House* and had to put it aside as I was overloading on medical jargon.

No.7 Discovering blogging – I am enjoying this very much. Although I am not really doing anything that interesting I enjoy finding little things to write about. I am not sure whether this might be a catalyst to change direction in my career. I would still love to work with film-makers and make movies all over the world but I would also like to take it down a gear. I don't want to become a scriptwriter – that is a very special talent and when you have read as many bad scripts as I have you can really appreciate the talent when a good script comes your way. There is no doubt how you feel when you read a great script – I was lucky enough for Quentin Tarantino to send me two of his best scripts to read at a very early stage. They are unputdownable. I don't think I could get to that stage.

I also don't know what I would write about. You can't endlessly write about having cancer and going bald. That will be over soon.

No. 8 Being spoiled – I can really recommend this aspect. Apart from all the gifts and flowers and cards, etc. I have been cooked for, cleaned for, whims catered for, films screened for in private and (now that I have Esther) I am driven wherever I want to go and prevented from even emptying the dishwasher. I have to admit that I rather like it and could get used to it. I don't want to have full staff but I could definitely handle a housekeeper, a chauffeur and a butler at the very least.

I was hoping that my list might run to the tidy number of ten things good about cancer but I have run out of steam. Last session of FEC tomorrow. More after that and perhaps the last two good things. The bad things are pretty obvious and I really don't need to write about them.

Lost days

22 JULY 2013

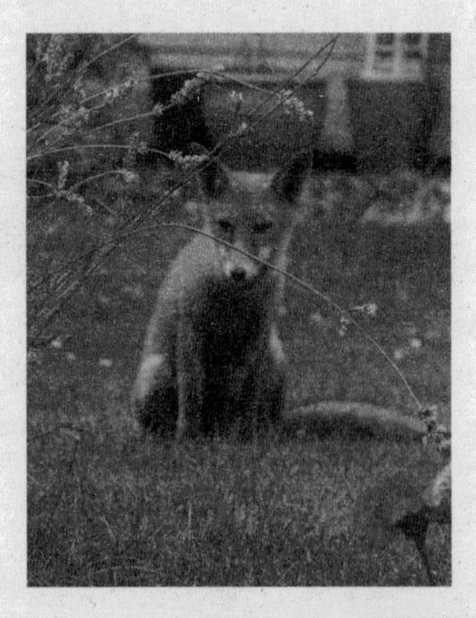

The fox who has moved into the house along with a blackbird and a pigeon. All very Springwatch *here*

I had my third round of chemo on Thursday, which means I am halfway through. It was the last dose of the three powerful cytotoxic chemo drugs called FEC: Fluorouracil, Epirubicin and Cyclophosphamide. Two of these are given by slow injection at the same time as a saline drip, via a cannula into a vein. My veins are already pretty shot (I could never be a serious drug addict) and so the only place they could find a viable vein was by my left elbow. The Epirubicin is the one which is the same colour as a Berocca drink, the Fluorouracil is colourless and is actually the smallest of the three but also the most painful and the last one is given as a drip. The whole process takes a couple of hours.

And so we bid farewell to the chemo combo and from the next time onwards I will only have one drug: Docetaxel. This one, though, requires you to take steroids all the way through. I know that steroids are a wonder drug but they really are awful things. You swell up like a helium balloon and feel completely pumped up. I can't imagine how we missed noticing that those East German female shot-putters in the seventies were on steroids. I already look like a tougher version of them. In fact, Esther pointed out that with my bald head and my white vest I wouldn't have looked out of place at the English Defence League rally this weekend. Thanks.

The day after chemo I felt almost human. The main feeling is like a woozy jet lag. You feel slightly out of sorts and out of your body and also nauseous. Nausea is awful. It must be horrible being nauseous when you are pregnant – at least I can take pills for it. However, the next two days are a blur. Even listening to *Test Match Special* exhausted me. By Day 4 I had had enough. You know that feeling when wherever you lie in bed you feel uncomfortable and everything is a huge effort and quite frankly you have just had about as much as you can take? That's when the local wildlife decided to put on a show for me. I was lying there feeling a little bit sorry for myself and Esther was watching telly when she noticed the fox inside the lounge. I think he feels left out as he sees the cat coming in and out and also the odd pigeon who makes his way into the house and clearly he wanted to see what all the fuss was about. I took the photo earlier of him this year in the garden – I just missed him and the cat having a chat.

Last night Grably started to play-bite me – he doesn't draw blood and it doesn't hurt. I think he is just practising for when I do die and he is forced to eat me as he can't open the cat food pouches on his own. For now he is saved as I am up and about today – for at least an hour or two. The one great advantage of having cancer is I am still hypothermic (34 degrees today) so I can lie in this heat under a duvet and still 'feel the benefit'.

Weighty issues

26 JULY 2013

I went a bit Pollyanna last week with my good things about cancer. Remember Pollyanna? I identified with her because she too was Titian-haired... I was never as good or as positive about life as she was. I suspect the book is massively out of vogue now... after all, who wants to always look on the Bright Side of Life when there's the misery of reality TV and the worldwide economic meltdown to cheer us up?

But I digress. I am fed up with chemo. I am not sure if the phrase comes from feeling sick after eating too much: which is appropriate as chemo really makes you feel sick even when you are hungry. My grandmother who was Hungarian struggled to learn idiomatic

English and she took the phrases very literally. When she had eaten enough she would declare herself 'fed up'. I am told, but don't remember this, that one day when I was little my mother got a call from a garage pleading with her to come and collect my grandmother. Apparently she had seen the sign 'Self-Drive Hire' and so had hired a car and sat in it asking it to drive itself. I think I may have inherited some of her skewed logic – recently, when I was in Arizona, I got quite fixated by the 'Adopt a Highway' scheme where people or their pets, sporting clubs, etc., adopt a few miles of the motorway. One sign had me very intrigued: 'Escapees RV Club'. I asked at a gas station as to whether these were Vietnam veterans or Korean War vets . . . no, these are owners of recreational vehicles escaping their families.

So I am fed up with chemo. I am also fed up with the weight issue. Here I was thinking that the sallow-skinned, sunken-eyed, thin-as-a-rake look was chemo chic but it turns out that is heroin chic and chemo-chic is more Jabba the Hutt. Isn't it enough that we have to suffer all the other indignities but no, we also have to balloon in size? It doesn't seem fair as for at least one week out of every three I am too tired and too nauseous to eat. I exist on the occasional handful of anything that takes my fancy. Then the next two weeks I try to eat very healthily and take some exercise but yet every time I go back to the hospital I have put on weight.

Before poisoning you the hospital has to take your measurements – weight and height, etc. – as they work out to the exact millimetre your surface area and that determines how much poison your veins will take. So every time I try and bribe the nurses to under-report they refuse on the grounds that I might miss out on a drop of toxin. It can't all be steroids. As Esther just pointed out – she spent a week in hospital nil by mouth and still came out the same weight. I have been relatively incensed by comments about Kate Middleton's baby tummy and yet no one is highlighting the issue of chemo tummy. Maybe that will be my new campaign... I think the ribbon should be a yellowy green colour – something sallow or vomity. Perhaps Farrow & Ball have a suitable paint palette.

It's one thing to deal with the weight problem but I am also struggling to know how to deal with the bald head. It's not as simple as saving on shampoo. I have some small areas of hair and I seem to get rashes either from wearing hats or traumatized hair follicles. I am now exfoliating my head in the shower. If anyone has any suggestions I would be very grateful. Perhaps it's a kind of cradle cap like babies get?

On the wildlife front we have been relatively undisturbed these last few days. I made an appearance in the garden yesterday which probably satisfied the flora and fauna of North London for a while so they don't have to come in and see for themselves that I am extant.

Ribbons and nose hair

28 JULY 2013

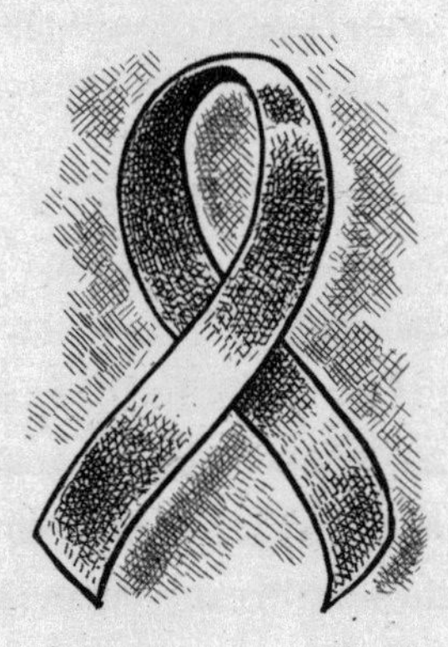

One of the things about having cancer is you become aware of all the great charities pushing for awareness and cures and research into cancer. So many of their names are familiar from the high-street charity shops. In our high street we have Marie Curie and Cancer Research alongside the familiar names like Oxfam and Scope. I don't know how many people are involved in working for the charities or how many people are working in the research field. We have a cousin who was working for the Marie Curie Institute and is now at a government-funded lab – he is, as I understand it, a geneticist working on the genome code looking for the rogue cancer code. I think.

I remember when I first became aware of the genome code. I hope I spelt that correctly. It's 2 a.m. as I write unable to sleep so I could well be writing in Cyrillic... Anyway, I was on a train returning to university after a trip home. The train I took from the North started in Scotland and ended in Devon. Inevitably, if I got on at home in York there would already be legions of drunk Scots and Geordies whatever time of the day or night it was, and if I got on at Bristol to go to York, it would be full of squaddies. If I was coming south from York I would bury my nose in a book, so old-fashioned I know, but this was the early eighties so no iPods, Kindles, and the Sony Walkman had only just been invented. If I was coming north I would, however, often play poker with the squaddies... but that's another story.

So there I was on a southbound train with my head buried in a bleak Russian novel when the chap opposite me engaged me in conversation. Now there are rules about transportation and conversation as far as I am aware. If a stranger beside you on a flight, or opposite you on a train, has their nose in a book that's a sign. A sign to not start chatting to them. But this chap was oblivious to the rules. The reason I answered back is that he was radiating excitement – not in a drug-fuelled kind of hyper-excitement but genuine, almost childlike, excitement, and just had to tell me why. As it turned out he was going to a university to present one of the earliest findings about the genome project. He was in some ways like Crick and Co. with the DNA helix. He was very confident that this would change EVERYTHING and that by the time I was forty there would be a database with everyone's mapped-out genetic code and cancers, etc., would almost be a thing of the past.

Where he is now or what happened in the intervening years since 1984 I have no idea. I don't yet have my mapped code (just as well, as I find remembering a four-digit pin code hard) and apparently there are 3.1 billion letters in the DNA code in every one of the 100 trillion cells in the human body and we have over 40,000 genes. There is no way I would remember my code.

I suppose the scientists have their work cut out and I can't be too cross that some twenty-nine years later the cure for cancer hasn't come from the genome work.

But back to raising awareness of cancers. Associated with breast cancer awareness is the pink ribbon campaign. Ribbons were used to raise awareness for the first time in the Iran hostage crisis (what happened after *Argo*'s credits rolled). The hostages were held from 1979 to 1981 and one of the relatives started tying yellow ribbons to trees outside her house, inspired by the song 'Tie a Yellow Ribbon to the Old Oak Tree' etc.

In the early eighties a red ribbon was first used to raise awareness of AIDS and HIV. In 1991 Evelyn Lauder of the Estée Lauder family and Alexandra Penney, editor-in-chief of *Self* magazine (I love that title), were inspired by Charlotte Hayley, someone with breast cancer who had worn a peach-coloured ribbon and decided to use a pink ribbon attached to the magazine. It is now recognized in over thirty countries. Evelyn, who had had breast cancer herself, also founded a cancer centre in the US for treatment and early diagnosis. She died in 2011 but Estée Lauder estimates that over $335 million has been raised towards research and that they have distributed over 80 million ribbons.

Staggering, isn't it?

October is Breast Cancer Awareness Month. And I am telling you all of this both because it would be lovely if you see a pink ribbon to buy one for me and others (they are £1) and also because the campaign is looking to slightly change direction or rather add a dimension. This year they want people not only to be breast aware but to be aware of what cancer does to family and friends as well as the patient. I have offered to help so watch this space for more info...

And now for something completely different, as Monty Python would say. Nose hair.

Up until now I have not loved nose hair. In fact, one man I worked with had such bad middle-age onset hair growth from nose and ears they virtually formed a moustache. At Christmas I did consider buying him clippers or a lawnmower, anonymously of course. Anyway, I was not especially fond of mine and vaguely worried that it might show. Now that I don't have any I think I have discovered the reason for it. This is not a scientific discovery to rival said genome project, but more of an observation. Without nasal hair I drip. Like a small child. Yet another glorious side effect of this toxic lifestyle. Now aren't you glad I chose a pink ribbon picture rather than a nasal hair shot?

Thumbs up to A & E

1 AUGUST 2013

I have been very lucky (aside from getting cancer, that is) to be treated by the NHS in the superlative Macmillan Cancer Centre so this week I decided to treat myself to another version of the NHS and visit A & E. I have had some embarrassing trips in the past to the emergency rooms of hospitals, haven't we all... Please don't get me wrong – I haven't had to have a hamster removed from my private parts but I have had some stupid accidents.

I don't know whether your mother told you this, but mine said I should always have clean knickers on even if I haven't actually bathed just in case I have to go to hospital. When I was doing up my first flat and painting all hours of the day and night I forgot this rule. I managed to spill Nitromors in my eye whilst stripping a wooden window frame and only realized as we were pulling into the hospital that I had last night's knickers on. Despite crying with pain and having an eyeball so swollen and red that I looked like I had gone several rounds with Rocky Balboa, I insisted that my friend drive me home to get fresh pants. By the time we got to A & E they were pretty cross that I hadn't come sooner to get the acid flushed out. I explained about the knickers. They accepted the explanation but did say it was unusual for eye patients to strip down to their underwear.

So on Monday I had on nice fresh silk underwear (just in case) and toddled off to the emergency room. With an embarrassingly trivial issue. I had trapped the thumb of my right hand in the back door, letting my cat out at dawn. On Friday. By Saturday it was swollen and throbbing. By Sunday it was red hot and by Monday it was the colour of under-ripe lime with a lot of hot red lines going down my wrist.

As I have mentioned before, Greg is very good in the emergency room waiting area as he can juggle and do Donald Duck voices but I now have a trump card: cancer. I flashed bald head and chemo card and was immediately whisked off into a room by myself just in case any of the sick people had chickenpox (which in chemo patients manifests as shingles) or a cold (pneumonia) or were generally feverish. Having no immunity means that a simple bruise becomes a septic blood clot. Still, it was pretty embarrassing to hold up my thumb to two wonderfully easy-on-the-eye young male doctors. One was Lebanese and an obstetrician doing a two-week rotation in A & E for some variety. I would have happily succumbed to a pelvic examination if required and also I had on the nice pants. The other was half Italian, half Irish, and a delightful full-time A & E doctor. They were very nice and quite excited as they hadn't had a chemo patient to play with. They had to draw blood and get it tested – haemoglobin levels and platelets and also liver and kidney functions and they knew they couldn't give me any ordinary antibiotics because of the chemo. The blood work took forty-five minutes but they filled in the time nicely by X-raying my thumb. I jumped to the head of the queue in front of a man who looked like his arm was hanging out of its socket. I felt smug and deeply embarrassed. Lucky for me the bald head meant he couldn't complain.

After ascertaining that my thumb was not broken and that my bloods were OK the operation commenced. The Irish/Italian doctor explained that the thumb is a complex digit. I knew that opposable thumbs were a must in higher evolutionary terms but I didn't realize just how special they are. If I have got this right – and I was distracted a bit by his beauty – our thumbs are on backwards in terms of the tendons and the nerves and it is the only digit that we can bend in pretty much any direction. So it took a bit of time to numb it and then lance the septic wound and I was given a plaster and some antibiotics and sent home.

Both Em and Esther wanted to come with me but arriving with an entourage for a thumb injury was too much. If I had sliced off the thumb or needed to have an ingested hamster removed I would've taken them.

So thumbs up to Royal Free A & E.

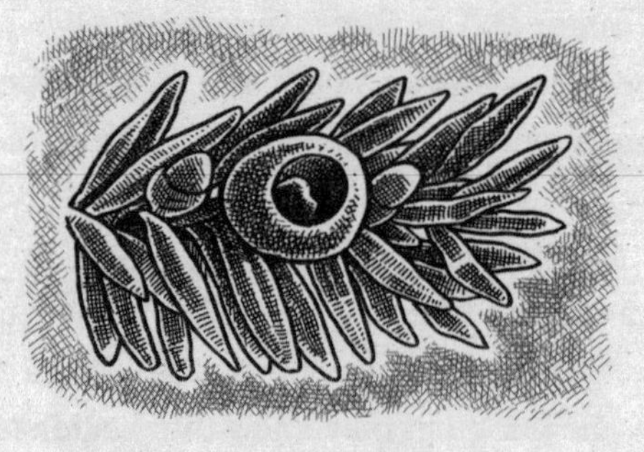

My next chemo is tomorrow morning. It's a new regime called Docetaxel which is from yew trees. Yew trees are highly poisonous and planted almost exclusively in churchyards as they have been associated with death for centuries. This doesn't bode well. The side effects of this drug are very pronounced and I have to take a lot more steroids. I am already feeling like an East German shot-putter so not looking forward to more pumping up.

Having said that, yew trees are fascinating. The oldest one in this country is in Perthshire and is called the Fortingall Yew and is estimated to be between 2,000 and 4,000 years old. The oldest yew in the world is in Spain at Bermiego Asturias and is called the Teixu l'Iglesia (English yew) and is over 4,000 years old. The yew is believed to be a guide to the land of shadows, a harbinger of death. Its wood was used by the English longbowmen (the two-fingered insult comes from them too). In 1021 the yew was first used to treat cardiac symptoms and by the mid-twentieth century to manufacture chemo drugs. So two fingers up to chemo.

Let's hope I get the longevity side effect and not the other.

More another day.

Fourth round chemo

9 AUGUST 2013

It is with a certain amount of trepidation that you head to the hospital on the chemo day. I was a little more apprehensive due to the new drug and also the steroids whizzing through my body. But of course everything was fine.

My oncologist thinks the tumour has shrunk again and is pleased with progress. I see the onco-plastic surgeon on 27 August when we will discuss the surgery in November and they will measure the tumour again.

The new drug was very cold and relatively painless. The most painful part of the process is putting in the cannula and finding a vein. My veins used for the last three chemos have collapsed – that means that they have basically gone flat and the blood pushes hard to get through thus making them like long bruises. When I raise my hands higher than my ears it aches and is very painful. If I reach for a glass or a plate in my eye-level kitchen cupboards I cry out in pain. I wasn't expecting this. I can't have my blood pressure test done on my arms any more – the cuff has to be put on my lower leg. The fourth chemo egress was through my right hand. By the time we get to 6 it could be through my eyeballs.

All went well and my reward for being a good patient was to have John do reflexology and Reiki on me.

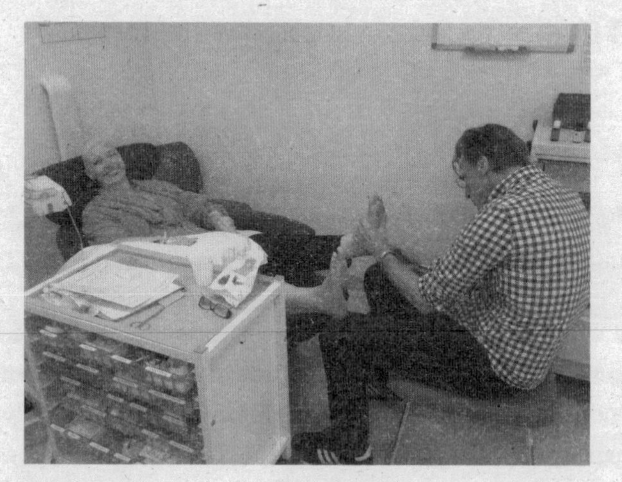

Then last night Em, Esther and I went to see *The Book of Mormon*, which was a fantastic way to end the day. I highly recommend it.

So far no adverse side effects bar the fizzing steroids which make sleeping staccato. I am told that I will start feeling side effects by Day 4 – the most common is aching muscles and bones for about two weeks. I dive into neutropenia on Day 5 this time and it lasts for ten days. I should expect migraines, swollen ankles, burning feet and hands and discoloured painful nails. Esther thinks I should hide them with black nail polish so we will post pictures of me as a Goth.

The agony and the ecstasy…

15 AUGUST 2013

Actually, there is nothing ecstatic about this taxane yew tree poisoning, it is all agony. Perhaps the ecstasy will come after this agony is over.

I am in pain. Every single muscle, tendon and bone aches. It is like the flu times ten or going twelve rounds with Mike Tyson, Muhammad Ali and Joe Bugner in a tag team. It came on Sunday and doesn't appear to be abating at all. I was warned that I could have some pain but for f***'s sake, I am being treated in a hospital. Can't I be given morphine? No – you are told to take paracetamol. That doesn't seem fair. If I can be poisoned by top-of-the-range drugs can't I have really fancy painkillers?

I will post more when I am a little bit more together. But for now a thought on paracetamol:

Why is there no aspirin in the jungle? Because the parrots-eat-'em-all…ouch!

There's no ecstasy yet…

21 AUGUST 2013

Sorry not to have posted for a while but as you will have guessed this chemo knocked me for six. It wasn't just the excruciating pain, it was the throat and mouth full of ulcers that made drinking water feel like swallowing razor blades, but also the usual side effects of fatigue, etc., that meant I could barely walk, talk, let alone blog.

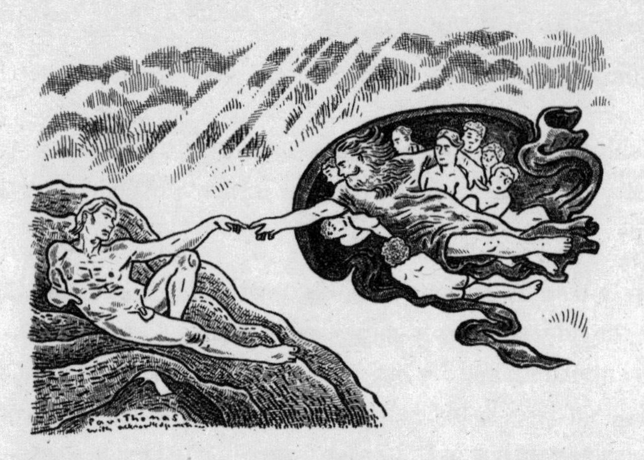

The Creation of Adam, with acknowledgements to Michelangelo

I can hardly compare myself to Michelangelo whose agony was to lie on his back and paint the Sistine Chapel at the Vatican – it took him over four years to paint the frescoes there. The title of today's blog is inspired by the film *The Agony and the Ecstasy*, starring the NRA poster boy Charlton Heston, where the ecstasy appears to be a personal battle with Leonardo to prove who was the better painter (Hollywood licence). When I was at university, in my holidays I worked as a tour guide in Europe, so I had taken parties of Americans around the chapel, most had barely heard of Michelangelo and I fear most left there thinking it was Charlton Heston who painted it. We were always told that the centre part of the ceiling, representing Genesis, depicted God giving life to Adam. Then one day Vincenzo was there taking a group that included a brain surgeon. The brain surgeon pointed out that the cloak that God is wrapped in is a very specific shape, exactly like a cross-section of the brain, and the random green flag fluttering below was in fact the cerebral cortex. Look at it closely – he was right. God is not giving Adam life. He is giving him knowledge and reasoning. Cool, huh? If only the same could be said about Heston... he seems to have left reasoning at the altar of gun-toting madness.

But enough about dead painters. I have to be brutally honest, this chemo was just not fun. The hospital had mentioned (almost as an afterthought) that there might be some pain associated with this poisoning. SOME PAIN, that's British understatement for you. It was agonizing. Every muscle, tendon, bit of skin screamed out and the pain was like little electric shocks shuddering through my body. I haven't been through childbirth, nor have I ever broken anything (apart from the rib and infamously my jaw) so I can't compare it to those levels of pain. All I know is that I am not a wuss but this was very real and awful. As previously posted, the doctor suggested paracetamol. My arse. Didn't even take the edge off.

By the time Greg got back from Scotland I couldn't speak or swallow (ulcers) and I was writhing around in agony. Poor Esther and Em had had to watch me being altogether rather pathetic. Greg went into Superman mode (although he kept his underwear inside his pants) and marched off to the pharmacy to sit with the pharmacist on his computer and work out the strongest cocktail of over-the-counter drugs that I could take alongside the chemo. For seven days I was on no solids, very little liquids but a steady diet of maximum-strength co-codamol, Nurofen and paracetamol. I also had novocaine for the ulcers and my GP very sweetly organized for me to get something else for them, and so after ten days I have emerged out of my chrysalis – not as a butterfly but as a pain-free bald blimp.

This chemo has also seen off the last of my hair. I am hanging onto the remaining five eyelashes in the right eye. I have tried mascara and a lengthening gel and my last resort will be superglue. Losing these means that I do now feel like a cancer patient. Bald, eyelashless, retaining water and listing slightly in my gait.

Esther has meanwhile turned into Martha Stewart – although with the liberal use of swear words she is channelling Martha the jailbird, rather than Martha the wholesome. She arrived having knitted me a wonderful beanie and has since embarked upon knitting another one. I have no knitting skills and as far as I can see it involves starting, unpicking, starting again, swearing, unpicking and more swearing. The result is a fabulous cotton hat. I am now slightly worried that she will be pickling all sorts of things for the harsh winter months. She has already tidied up my fridge, my kitchen drawers, and is about to embark on my study. As you know, I file by stacking papers up randomly on any available surface. Post-cancer I could become very organized: a slightly frightening thought for those who know me well.

This poison has other new side effects not yet experienced by me. Swelling and water retention – really galling considering I have hardly eaten – and also skin rashes that bleed. On top of that the palms of my hands have become hot and itchy. And no, I haven't been having fun on my own... At first I got really excited when the right hand started, being told that that is a sign you are coming into money. I assume this comes from the idea that if someone itches their palm in front of you they are looking for a tip – waiters, etc. famously did it to elicit money from customers. I gather that the left palm itching means you will be giving money away. Given that both itch I guess any money I give away I will get back which means I will break even... phew.

Whilst lying there, itching, bleeding from suppurating wounds (slight exaggeration there), tossing and turning in agony, I fantasized about what my first meal might be. I fixated on Indian food – a gorgeous creamy sag paneer with rice and dal; then Mexican – a burrito washed down by a margarita; a healthy Vietnamese Pho soup; a stir-fry – mostly by walking down our high street in my brain. As it turned out my first solids were a small spoonful of Ambrosia Creamed Rice Pudding and half a baked potato. Not quite so exotic.

Again, cancer reduces you to banality. I have studiously avoided books on cancer experiences but a friend did send me a graphic novel called *Cancer Vixen* by Marisa Acocella, a Manhattan graphic artist. She is the *Sex and the City* cancer girl. Her treatment involved her not losing her luscious locks and always going to chemo in her Jimmy Choos. I heard yesterday that Cate Blanchett is going to play her in the film from the book. That's bloody typical. Where are the heroines without hair, eyebrows and eyelashes? I bet if the film had been based on my blog she wouldn't have done it. Em of course did the real portrayal in *Wit* – which Mike Nichols directed. An incredibly powerful and moving (aka upsetting) story of courage and cancer. She shaved her head . . .

On a final – rather weird – note. There is a huge police operation here in the UK looking into decades of child abuse by a now-dead DJ and the police have called it 'Operation Yew Tree'. I now understand why. It's because yew tree poison is toxic and painful and destructive. Salutary thought. I wonder if they did that intentionally?

Living without

25 AUGUST 2013

Having cancer means I have to have chemo (yuck) and having chemo means I have to do without several things.

There are some things not essential to life as we know it. Unless you are a hairdresser you don't need curling tongs, straighteners, heated rollers, shampoo and conditioner or visits to the hairdresser. I clearly don't need any of these things at the moment but weirdly I do miss some of the rituals associated with getting ready. Showers that used to take me a leisurely amount of time are now functional and take five minutes max. Since the only body hair that is tenaciously clinging to life is a small patch on my legs below my calf muscles, I only need to shave these areas from time to time. I estimate that over the course of a month I am saving myself at least forty-five minutes in the shower by not shaving. Not having to wash, rinse, condition and rinse your hair every other day probably saves me ninety minutes a month. So what do I do with this new-found two hours and fifteen minutes – nothing much. I do ponder about other losses which are not so easy.

I have lost my sense of taste. I have what's called 'metal mouth'. Not like Madonna's new-found dental prosthetics, this side effect is all about taste. Since I haven't spent much time in my life sucking on coins or biting down on a bit like a horse, I am not sure that the taste I have is metallic. It feels more like a mouthful of old seawater. It tastes slightly salty and makes everything taste the same. Even without so many ulcers (still have the pesky blighters in my throat) I am finding food a bit challenging. I like spices, which in turn hurt the ulcers. I like salt, ditto, and I hope that ice cream will relieve the ulcers and give me a sweeter-tasting mouth, but alas, that's a pipe dream – presumably a metallic pipe. So it looks as though I will have whale breath through all the chemo. Yum . . . who wants a kiss?

Another painful thing to live without are eyelashes. This is not just vanity, although that is probably the honest reason that I am mourning their loss. But eyelashes do have a function. Aside from keeping dirt, etc., out of the eye, they also keep moisture in. Now I look as though I am permanently upset. I also see double and that makes reading virtually impossible. Apparently the loss of your eyelashes is called 'madarosis'. The average human has between 100 and 150 on their upper eyelid. No wonder my last remaining five look pathetic. It takes approximately seven to eight weeks for them to grow back. Which means that I may have them in time for Christmas. Forget my front teeth, Santa, I want long luscious eyelashes like a camel.

Similarly eyebrows. They do have a function to prevent sweat and water from streaming down our faces into our eyes. Neanderthal man had a more pronounced forehead with a kind of ridge that protected his eyes until he developed eyebrows. Maybe my body will adapt along similar evolutionary lines and next time you see me I will have grown an awning above the eye socket.

Yet another weird loss due to alopecia is I can't get goosebumps. They are formed at the base of the hair follicle and involuntarily your hair stands on end because you are scared or cold. It is a reflex. The same thing happens to animals. They puff up their fur both to create warmth and insulation but also to look bigger and give themselves confidence when they are scared. In almost every language this reaction is called by something to do with poultry. In French it is '*chair de poule*'. I do also like the story that in seventeenth-century London syphilis was referred to as being bitten by the Winchester Goose. A reference to the prostitutes licensed by the Bishop of Winchester around his London palace. But since I am not familiar with syphilis I don't know whether you get goosebumps or not. I don't as I don't have body hair. Without eyebrows and the ability to get goosebumps how will you know when I am scared? And without eyelashes how will you know if I am upset or just leaking? Hmm, a conundrum. I can't get false goosebumps but I can get false eyelashes and eyebrows. Maybe that will be the next step.

What I have gained through cancer (apart from the support and love of friends and family, etc. etc.) is chemo brain. It really is a medical fact. It's like pregnancy brain. Emma C. thinks it's for a reason that I can't read or watch films or do anything – that it is my body which is making my brain shut down so I am only able to concentrate on healing. Whatever the reason for it I think I may need to carry a notebook at all times. So when something pops into my head I write it down. It will cut down on unnecessary trips into the kitchen, basement, etc., when I stand there and for the life of me have no idea why I am there. On the other hand, with blurred vision I might not be able to read my handwriting and still stand there like an idiot. I think the answer might be to carry a tape recorder (an old-fashioned idea but I can't think of what they are called now) and record my thought and play it back. I am not sure that that will work either since I am liable to forget I recorded something. Again a conundrum.

Whilst I remember, I am seeing the onco-plastic surgeon on Tuesday to discuss surgery and learn about implants and false nipples and then I am being blasted with chemo on Thursday. So lots to look forward to . . . if I remember.

Chemo the Fifth

30 AUGUST 2013

And gentlemen in England now a-bed
Shall think themselves accursed they were not here,
And hold their manhoods cheap whiles any speaks
That fought with us upon Saint Crispin's day.

Henry V, Shakespeare

It seems appropriate to have Henry V's rallying cry at Agincourt for the last chemo. Hurrah for Harry, England and St George.

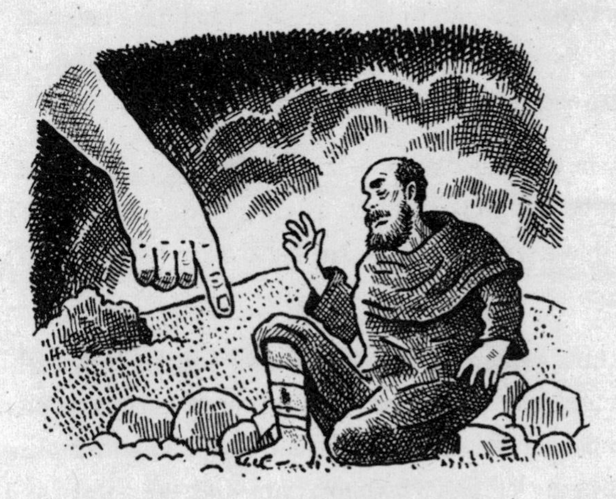

St Peregrine, patron saint of cancer

Talking of saints, I discovered recently that the patron saint of cancer is called St Peregrine, who was a thirteenth-century monk from Italy. In his devotion he always stood, and in later life developed varicose veins and cancer of the leg. The doctors decided to amputate and the night before the operation he dreamed that Christ descended from the cross and touched his leg and he was cured. He lived well into his eighties. Lucky bastard didn't need chemo. I might try the same trick before my next nuking.

I had a preliminary meeting with the onco-plastic surgeon on Tuesday. She has had a sense of humour bypass but I suppose it is better to wish for a good surgeon than a comedy genius. She didn't have any of my paperwork and didn't know if the tumour had shrunk but the good news is that the surgery will either be three or four weeks after my last chemo, so either on 21 or 28 October with radiotherapy starting around my birthday in mid-November. Which means that this whole experience could be behind me by the end of this calender year. We still don't know if it will be a mastectomy or a lumpectomy. Either way I have been told not to look at photos on the Internet until after next chemo as it may put me off. Not a good sign, methinks.

When she examined me she did find a new lump. I cannot believe that my body is growing anything when I am being poisoned in this way. I guess it is defiant. So she booked me in for an ultrasound and biopsy.

First thing yesterday Greg and I went into the hospital for the ultrasound and biopsy. The morning didn't start particularly well as I grabbed a herbal tea and the cup exploded, with boiling water drowning my left hand. It almost immediately blistered and had to be dressed. You are not supposed to come into hospital and injure yourself. That's just not playing by the rules.

It was Greg's first time at chemo and all of the nurses went into a complete flutter and he didn't even have to show off his juggling skills.

The scan showed two new cysts, one in each breast, which were aspirated... a large needle is inserted and the fluid (aka pus) is drained off. Yummy. Then they biopsied the new lump in my left breast. Again a huge needle is inserted and it has a kind of claw on the end to grab some cells. Not fun. The results, however, were to be given within thirty minutes so at least it would be quick. However, about ten minutes later the staff nurse came down with the bad news... I had slithered off the petri dish and it had to be done all over again. I think they just wanted to see Greg again and manufactured the slithering story to cover themselves. So back I went to be stabbed all over again. This time I didn't slither and the biopsy showed that this is just another fibroadenoma and not cancer.

After that we saw the oncologist and the pharmacist and I left with enough drugs to open my own pharmacy. Sadly no morphine, but something to act as a preventative measure for the debilitating ulcers and also codeine for the pain.

Esther joined us for lunch in the hospital roof gardens and then John appeared later to be my personal reflexologist and Reiki healer. The chemo nurses thought all their Christmasses had come at once. John and Greg certainly brought up the woof factor on the second floor.

I have organized a film premiere for the lovely staff with the help of Medicinema and my friend the über-PR guru Peter. Medicinema is a fantastic charity that is building cinemas in hospitals – with spaces for beds and wheelchairs and machines that go ping. They also programme the films. It is a wonderful distraction for long-term patients and gets them off the wards. Their latest venue is at Guy's Hospital and opens in November and I hope they will be able to get one at UCH where I am being treated. All the staff at the

Macmillan Centre are so excited as they very rarely get treats. Em will host the film which is called *The Love Punch*. She and Pierce Brosnan star in it – it is a caper/rom-com and looks fun. Another friend is working on champagne for the staff so all in all it should be a wonderful night. I won't be able to go as it is too soon after my next chemo.

On another note of self-aggrandizement, I think I mentioned the amazing work of Estée Lauder and the breast cancer awareness campaign. This October the campaign is changing its emphasis from not only being breast aware but how a diagnosis affects family and friends as well as the patient. They are running an article on me and my circle in *You* magazine sometime during that month so we were interviewed by the journalist for it. Greg and Esther were also interviewed. Greg described me as looking 'wrinkly' when I was in pain. Not sure he can be forgiven for that one. It's almost as bad as my ex, John, describing me as 'ample' in an interview with *Maxim* magazine. Not that I hold grudges, of course.

So here I am steroided up and waiting for the crash, which I expect will happen by Sunday. Hopefully the pain won't be as bad this time as my body has experienced this toxin once already. Fingers crossed. I look up steroids which I know are a miracle drug but do make me feel ruddy and bloated (not wrinkly). My steroid is called Dexamethasone which I have nicknamed Dexy's Midnight Runner. It is an anti-inflammatory with immunosuppressant properties (not sure why I need this last one as I am already immuno-compromised) and is twenty-five times more powerful than cortisol which is what your body produces in a morning to get you out of bed. That might account for some of my hyperactivity and spring-cleaning that I felt with the first dose. On the downside, aside from the bloating and swelling, it gives you very intense hot flushes.

Luckily Esther brought me a fan from her trip to the Alhambra so I can pretend just to be practising flamenco as I turn the shade of an overripe tomato.

Thank you, everyone, for your lovely wishes and thoughts. A lady I met through chemo who has been one cycle ahead of me is a real inspiration. Her name is Dorthe – she is from Denmark. Her breast cancer is very aggressive and she has three children under nine. If she can do this with so much grace then there is no reason that I can't get through this and one more cycle. The hard thing for me is saying goodbye to the last of my eyelashes. I am going to experiment with falsies before my photo is taken for the article. I fully expect to look like RuPaul on a bad day.

Spoke too soon

4 SEPTEMBER 2013

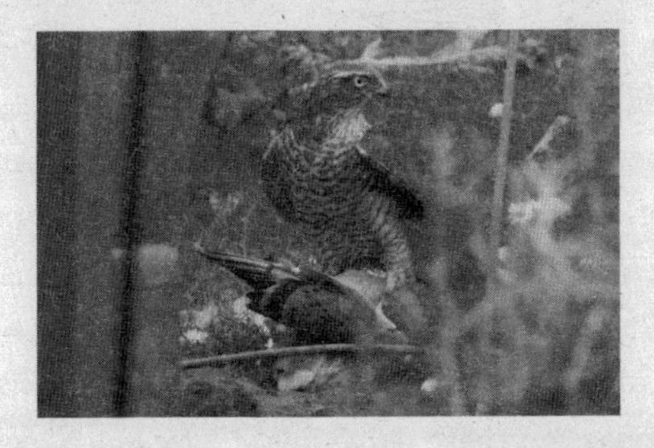

Wildlife update – sparrowhawk in garden attacking pigeon

I was rather too gung-ho and a wee bit pretentious to use Henry V's rallying cry when of course I still had to get through this fifth round of chemo and still have another blasting on 19 September, as well as get through the effects of that.

I am on Day 92 of 127 days of chemo. I didn't think that I would get this far when I started out. So I can be forgiven for jumping the gun to get to the end of this process. At the beginning I never thought about the seriousness of cancer and I certainly didn't dwell on the statistics or even the whole reality of a cancer diagnosis but lately there seems to have been so much press about cancer survival rates that it has crept into my consciousness. Don't worry, I am not getting maudlin or depressed, but I am a little surprised at my whole ostrich-like reaction.

I heard a programme on Radio 4 this week about breast cancer and tamoxifen. The side effects of this drug, which I am scheduled to take for ten years after I complete my chemo and surgery, sound as awful as this current poison. Apart from the ubiquitous violent hot flushes, muscle and joint ache, there are some other lovely little traits . . . like completely removing libido, etc. Blimey. I really don't want to be in pain, hot and disinterested in sex for a decade. Especially after having had a boob removed. There must be an alternative. The statistics suggest that the survival rate post-breast cancer without tamoxifen seems to halve. Currently the survival rates for someone of my age with my cancer for a year are good – 90 per cent, over five years this drops to about 80 per cent and then ten years to around 75 per cent. That all sounds good since of course I may be run over by a bus tomorrow (unlikely unless it is diverted through my bedroom, but you know what I mean). Without tamoxifen these percentages look much worse. I think I may actually finally have to become proactive and question the medical route being suggested of ten years of tamoxifen and look into alternatives. Up until now I haven't questioned the wisdom of the doctors but long-term I might just do so.

And I am feeling a little more rebellious about having to have the last chemo. I had assumed that my body would be better prepared for the side effects but despite that I still nosedived into pain and neutropenia. The ulcers came back with a vengeance and by Thursday I really couldn't swallow anything – even water was like razor blades in my throat. I asked Esther to get a doctor.

Since starting the chemo I have moved doctor's surgery to a lovely little practice round the corner. When Esther explained that I was neutropenic and needed a home visit they jumped into action. Sadly, they couldn't manage the home visit but did offer to slot me in at the end of the morning when there were no patients left and they could put me in a room which they would sterilize. The doctor was a locum – an eccentric chap who patted me on the head and told me that soon all of this would be a distant memory. He looked in my throat and then insisted that Esther take a look. Perhaps for a second opinion – after all, she had wanted to become a doctor when she was little. The ulcers were indeed large and angry, so he prescribed antibiotics and more mouthwash, etc., and even gave us his mother's chicken soup recipe. He asked me if I had eaten at all and was appalled when I said I had managed some mashed potato – that's for Germans, he said. What you need is protein and chicken soup is the best.

Armed with a whole new medicine cabinet of drugs I am hoping that I will start to feel better very soon. The antibiotics seem to have already started to work on the ulcers but the swallowing is still a major challenge. The aches and pains are subsiding and I may even get out for a walk this weekend. I am fed up with the cure being the worst part of this cancer experience.

On another note, a friend from Australia had been uncharacteristically quiet. She hadn't understood that I was going through lots of chemo, etc., and that it wasn't fun. Then her beagle got cancer and he is having chemo. Now she gets it. I hope he doesn't lose his fur. It must be horrible to be an animal in this situation – they don't understand that what is being done to them is for their own good... Ah, hang on, neither do I.

Yoda and E.T.'s love child

10 SEPTEMBER 2013

Yes, it's finally come to this. The last eyelash has gone and I have a new side effect called, rather prosaically, 'hand and foot syndrome' – the palms of my hands are red as are the bits in between my fingers and it's sore and a cross between eczema and as though I was dyeing something without wearing gloves.

Without eyelashes I cry all the time... no, not depressed, this is merely my eyes leaking. When I wake up in the morning I look like a crustacean or a sea lizard as I have rings of salt around my eyes. The salt is of course affecting my skin and no matter how expensive the under-eye treatment is (and believe you me, I have some very expensive different brands) it is of no use. I did try to put on a little make-up but that mostly ends up in the bags under my eyes or halfway down my nose. I have a small amount of eyebrow left and it just looks as though I over-plucked. Bearing in mind Greg's comment about me looking wrinkly (not that I hold a grudge) I am shocked to see how much I now look like the love child of Yoda and E.T. I am a similar colour to E.T. and as wrinkly as Yoda. And wouldn't you just know that this is the moment I am having my photo taken . . . bugger.

I am going to experiment with false eyelashes and rely on the kindness of friends to alert me to them migrating into a moustache or mono brow. I did a little research on a chemo website and was recommended to try MAC. Let's see.

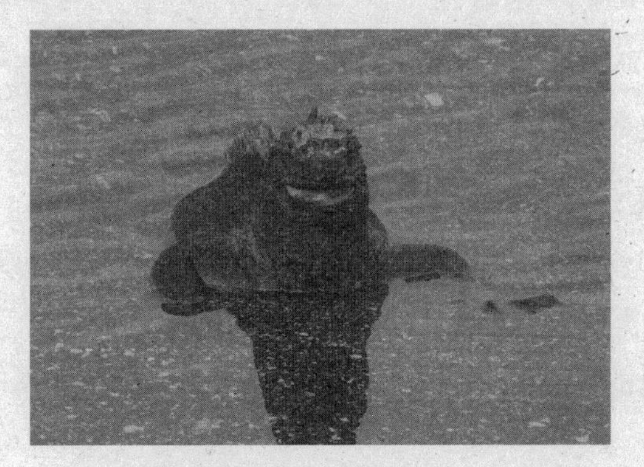

Me in the mornings

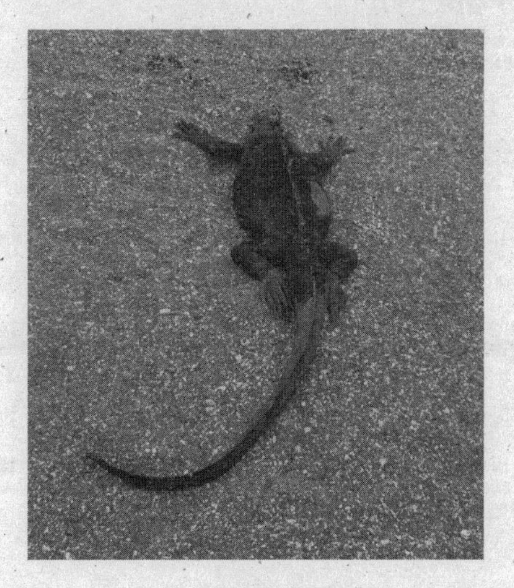

Me in the afternoons

I have a meeting with the surgeon on Tuesday and chemo again next Thursday. I really don't see the point of this last chemo. I am so very toxic even my palms are peeling. If the tumour has already shrunk (we hope) and I still need surgery and radiotherapy, what's the point of me suffering another three weeks of misery? I could use the time profitably – to grow back eyelashes (six weeks), hair (starts again four weeks after last chemo), other hair (no known time frame on that) and get myself into a more healthy position to face surgery. This makes sense to me . . . I hope the doctors agree.

For those of you following the wildlife update there was a greater spotted woodpecker on the bird feeder this morning. I felt a certain affinity with the headbanger as I do feel that this process can be a bit like banging your head against a brick wall.

Oh well, upwards and onwards.

To have or not to have . . .

17 SEPTEMBER 2013

I saw the surgeon today and it was pretty good news. The tumour has shrunk from 3.5 centimetres to 2 centimetres so they are confident that the surgery will be breast conservation. They will remove the tumour and about 1 centimetre around it and all lymph nodes in my armpit. Depending on the status of the invasive ductal carcinoma I may have to go back for a mastectomy. I will have to have radiotherapy. They promise that my breast will look normal but the nipple may be higher than its neighbour on the right. I will be a bit lopsided but not too much.

The doctors do want me to have the sixth chemo but I really don't want it as they will need to cut me open anyway. I have to make the decision by Thursday so I will spend tomorrow looking at the pros and cons and getting the medical opinion on Thursday when I see the oncologist. The team will have to give me empirical and medical evidence to proceed.

Thoughts welcome.

x

Chemo Number 6

18 SEPTEMBER 2013

I have decided that I don't want the sixth chemo and I want to try and take control of my body and this disease. I have many reasons for not wanting to do it – apart from the sheer hell that I will have to go through and the pain and the horrid side effects; if I don't have it then the surgery will be in four weeks which is much better. The radiotherapy will start three to four weeks after the surgery and I will hopefully get it all out of the way by 2014. I can't tell you how good it will feel to start the New Year with a very different aspect to the last seven months of 2013. I know I won't be in remission – that comes only after five years of being clear –but at least psychologically it will feel like a new start.

I know this is the right decision. I will give the oncologist a chance tomorrow to make a medical case for continuing with chemo. Since I am pretty sure that they won't be able to give me the cast-iron guarantee that the last chemo will make all the difference I am going to insist on not having it. Shirley, the staff nurse in the oncology department, did say that I might regret my decision if it comes back but let's face it, it won't be for me having done anything wrong. I have gone along with all the medical advice and have been a good patient. They refer to me as being 'pleasant' in all their correspondence with my GP, which is nice. I will still need to be cut open (at least once) and have radiotherapy so it's no walk in the park going forward but is at least all going to happen sooner.

I did a straw poll with my friends and family, most of whom are 100 per cent supportive. One friend who has been very close to cancer with her mum would prefer it if I let them finish the treatment but will support me and my decision.

Here's hoping.

I had a bit of a knock-back emotionally today. I had studiously avoided books and blogs on cancer but one book caught my eye and it's really wonderfully funny and evocative. It's called *The C-Word*, written by a twenty-eight-year-old called Lisa Lynch whose breast cancer was much more aggressive than mine. Imagine being twenty-eight – it's so unfair. Her book is very funny and I read it at the beginning of my treatment and dipped into it again today. I then decided to look at her blog and was blown away by the fact that she died in April this year. Her secondary cancer spread through her bones and into her brain and she died at only thirty-three years old. I am so lucky to be that much older. If you get the chance do look at her website – truly extraordinary person: www.alrighttit.blogspot.com.

Em treated me to my first catwalk show yesterday at London Fashion Week – we went to Maria Grachvogel's show. Her dresses and trousers are elegant and flowy – very fairy-tale gorgeous and made for women who are tall but who have hips and bottoms. They look so wonderful on Em but I am a little short for my weight and they swamp me, but it's nice to dream.

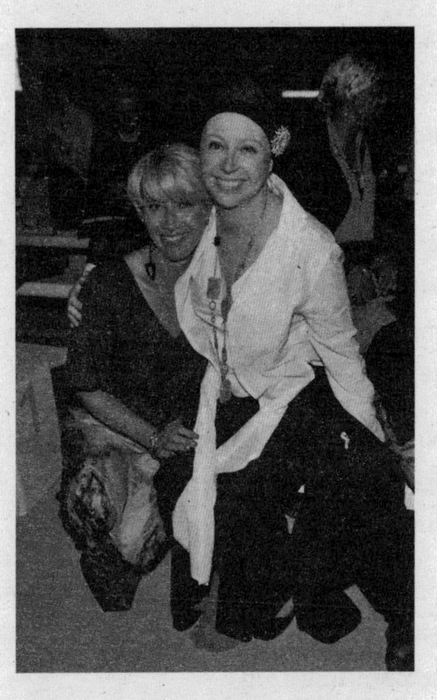

Em and me at Maria Grachvogel's London Fashion Week catwalk show yesterday. Her make-up artist gave me false eyelashes and eyebrows

Thank you, everyone, for the kind and loving messages – it's overwhelming to get such support.

I will let you know what the oncologist says tomorrow and whether I have had to capitulate to chemo or have been able to escape the last one.

Hurrah

19 SEPTEMBER 2013

I met with the oncologist today and they were 100 per cent supportive of me not having the sixth chemo and letting me get myself together for surgery. Surgery will be on 24 October and then radiotherapy in Nov/December.

I can't tell you how happy and relieved I am not to have been poisoned again today. In some respects chemo wasn't as bad as I feared – no wrapped around toilet bowl for hours vomiting, but that is the only side effect I didn't get.

I am beginning an immune-boosting diet from today which involves lots of turmeric, cruciferous veg and all sorts of supplements to rebuild my immunity.

I did skip out of the oncologist's room and whooped, until I saw a waiting room full of people who had to have chemo. I felt a little bad but couldn't help smiling a lot.

I have my photo shoot tomorrow for the Breast Cancer Awareness piece in *You* magazine. I am going to be bald and honest about what cancer and chemo does for you. I don't think I even want false eyelashes but may feel differently tomorrow.

Thanks for all the messages of support and love.

Chemo: 0, chest infection: 1

23 SEPTEMBER 2013

I escaped chemo on Thursday but went down with a chest infection on Friday night which almost hospitalized me. There really is some truth to the whole no-immunity issue. My guess is that someone sneezed on the Tube as we were going into the hospital and that manifested itself in problems with breathing.

Of course it all happened at the weekend. By Saturday morning I was having great difficulty breathing. I am an asthmatic so that only exacerbates the problem. I did get a house call from a GP through the NHS 111 system, which I thought had gone bust, but clearly it is a case of the postcode lottery and this time I am a winner.

The GP came within forty-five minutes and stayed for at least as long again. Initially they wanted to hospitalize me but I did my big sad eyes... don't send me to a place with sick people where I could pick up God knows what... so after checking my vitals and then putting me on a nebulizer (twice) and giving me steroids and antibiotics, they decided to leave me for a few hours and if I wasn't better I would have to go to hospital. Luckily I rallied a bit before the deadline so have been in bed ever since.

It is irritating. I feel like Sisyphus. I get to the top of the hill post-chemo and then find myself at the bottom again pushing a metaphorical boulder uphill.

Hopefully a combo of the immune-boosting diet and all the supplements, etc., I have invested in will start to pay dividends. I was supposed to see the nurse for a pre-surgery briefing today but as Esther pointed out it is probably not a good idea for me to go into a place full of immune-compromised people... I might infect someone else. It hadn't even occurred to me as so far everything is about me . . . me me me. Of course I should have thought that I could be a danger to others in similar situations. Clare Wise . . . licence to infect.

This appointment pre-surgery will give me details about how long I will be in hospital, etc. The surgery is scheduled for a Thursday – what is it about Thursdays? If I am going to have a bad day it is ALWAYS on a Thursday. At school it was double chemistry, double maths on Thursday afternoons. I am a Thursday's child who theoretically has far to go but in this case seems stymied by the curse of Thursdays. Chemo day was also Thursday and the day the raging ulcers came in was usually a week later on a Thursday. I think I even lost my job on a Thursday . . . neither parent died on a Thursday, which was considerate of them, but I have a sneaking suspicion that their funerals were Thursdays. When I am Queen – or Supreme Ruler – I will ban Thursdays, thus making a much easier transition to the weekend. I realize this would be a big shift for everyone who has got used to a seven-day week since the early Babylonian times some twenty-six centuries ago, but a change is as good as a rest for a blind bat, or something along those lines.

Ted Heath wanted a four-day week and then a three-day week in the troubled 1970s when we were hit by strikes and blackouts. I am in favour of a longer rest period these days but I suppose that's easy for me to say as I do little else but rest. The funny thing is that even though my weeks have no definition I still get excited by weekends and they do feel different.

This week, once I am better, I am going to get the wig cut so I look less like a regional newsreader. I will post pics of that for a laugh. I haven't worn the wig once – the summer was too hot and also the bloody thing is itchy and far too much. I might have to start wearing it now that it's getting colder, although Esther is knitting up a storm of hats for me.

The launch of Breast Cancer Awareness month

1 OCTOBER 2013

The lovely people at Estée Lauder invited me to the launch of Breast Cancer Awareness earlier this week. Evelyn Lauder had established the Breast Cancer Research Foundation in 1993 which to date has raised more than $450 million to help prevent and cure breast cancer in our lifetime. Her good work has been continued by her family and the company, who seem 100 per cent committed to making a success out of the BCA month.

The evening was hosted by the president of Estée Lauder and Elizabeth Hurley, who did a wonderful job of talking about the disease and also the research work that is going into early diagnosis and treatment as well as the groundbreaking work on my type of cancer – oestrogen-receptive environmentally caused tumours. She had attended a symposium at the Royal Marsden hospital with two professors and I will try and get more information about that as it sounded pertinent and fascinating.

The evening culminated with the lighting up of the BT tower in pink with a message running around the top about being breast aware. Do please look at the website www.BCAcampaign.com and even invest in a pink ribbon. Since 1994 the BCA campaign has donated over £30 million into research but each researcher's work costs around half a million so that doesn't end up going very far. They are funding medical research and clinical trials into an early phase cancer vaccine as well as improving ways to assess risk in young girls with family history.

There were three other women there who had all survived breast cancer and were in remission. Meeting women like this gives me great solace, not that I have ever thought I might be killed by this disease but it's still good to hear about survival.

I was introduced to Liz (as I now call her) at the exact moment I got one of those chemo-induced hot flushes where you literally start to run sweat in rivers down your whole body. She was very nice about me melting next to her and I worried that I might stain her immaculate look if I stood too close. I was reminded of a scene in *Sex and the City* in the last series when Samantha has cancer and is talking at a fundraiser and she gets one of those flushes and pulls off her wig and fans herself with it. I was very close to taking my Gloria Swanson hat off and doing the same. I hope my moist face doesn't show up on any of the photos that were taken that night.

Holiday

9 OCTOBER 2013

Sorry not to have posted anything for a while but I've been on holiday. It was wonderful on so many levels. Wonderful to be out of the flat – first time since diagnosis – and wonderful to be in the sun (Miami beach) and particularly wonderful to be surrounded by so many lovely people.

My friend Steph the polymath was celebrating his fiftieth with his oldest friend George in Miami. I didn't think I would be able to go what with the chemo, etc., but by cancelling the last chemo we were able to surprise him and join the week-long party. It felt so great to almost be normal – apart from being follically challenged and sweltering in 95-degree heat, with 90 per cent humidity and chemo-induced hot flushes every few minutes. Being the only bald woman in the hotel and in fact on the beach meant that everyone knew me and so when we left and said goodbye to our friends I also had to do a lap of the hotel staff.

Miami beach was beautiful and about thirty blocks away from the art deco area of South Beach (SoBe) and despite catching the edge of tropical storm Karen we were very lucky with blue skies and warm seas. It was great fun to be on holiday with fifty other people. I always had someone to play with, which of course took the pressure off Esther. I woke up early and sat at breakfast for at least three hours and was joined in the process by pretty much everyone. I felt like I was holding court, and indeed some would say I was. No wonder I came back very fat.

We had seen Steph two days before we left and I had basically lied to him about not being able to travel as I wanted to surprise him in Miami. We almost didn't make the surprise as Esther spotted him and Will at Heathrow and donned her hat and dove under a table, much to the amusement of the waiting staff. I was wandering around looking for a loo, so managed to miss the subterfuge. We got all the way to the hotel bar before seeing him again. He was very surprised and touched and even shed a tear or two. So the ruse worked.

The party was on the Thursday and came with a suckling pig on a spit roast, a stripper (who didn't actually strip), an Oompa-Loompa who handed out silly party wear and a man in a G-string serving 'cock'tails. All in all great fun and I even lasted till almost midnight. All the girls had booked into the hotel spa for a blowdry which apparently in America is called a 'blowout'. I also tried but for some reason they seemed to be fully booked, how ironic.

On that front, though, my hair is growing (seemingly coming through white). I still don't need a comb or shampoo but it won't be too long. The rest of my hair is coming back very patchy. Ankle hair, which has stayed all the way through chemo, is still growing and I have one or two pubes but still no eyelashes. When, oh, when will they come?

After Miami Esther and I rented a car and went to Key West for a few days. We visited the southernmost point of the US (only ninety miles to Cuba) and saw Ernest Hemingway's house and his six-toed cats (Esther wouldn't let me bring one back) and then had sundowners at Mallory Square. We had arrived on Key West's Oktoberfest so the place was brimming over with drunk students and the following day there was an unmistakable smell of vomit in the air. But we didn't let that spoil our time and found lovely places to eat.

We came home yesterday partied out and tired. I now need to cut back on the bingeing of alcohol and tasty but carb-heavy food and concentrate on getting myself into shape for surgery in a fortnight. Surgery will be 'breast conservancy' where they will cut out the lump and 2 centimetres of tissue all around it and take out all the nodes (lymph glands) in my left arm. Should they find anything else (spare lumps, more cancer or whatever else I keep hidden in there) then they might have to do the full mastectomy. I have no preference either way at the moment and will leave it in their hands. About three weeks after surgery I will embark on six weeks of radiotherapy which is around thirty minutes every day. I might as well move into the hospital.

I had some photos taken for Breast Cancer Awareness month by Charlotte Murphy for a *You* magazine article which will be out on 20 October. I begged the magazine not to use the cat photos as I didn't want to look like sad spinster with cat... and yet. Xxx

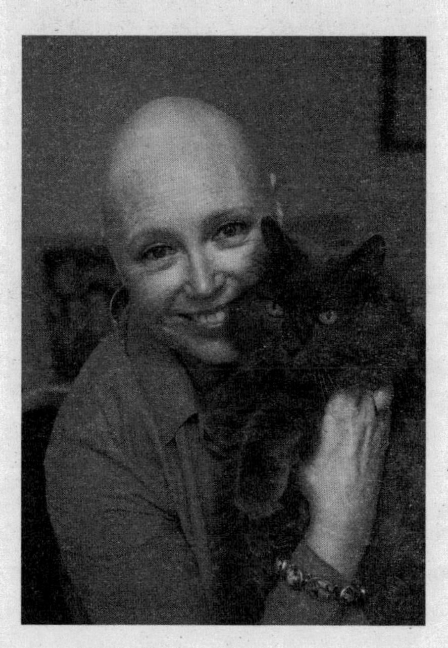

Lots of lovely comments

22 OCTOBER 2013

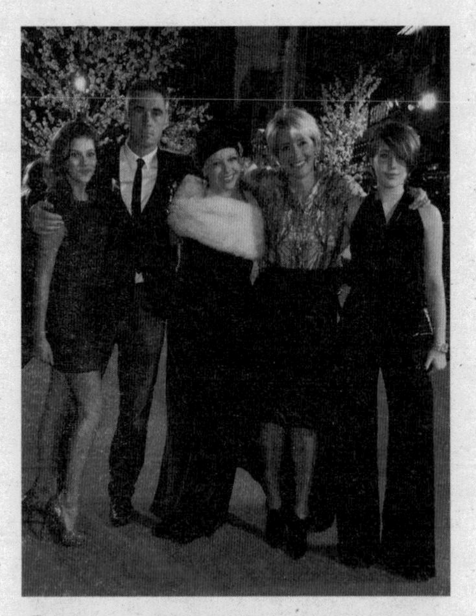

That's Lara (Gaia's friend), Greg (with pink ribbon), me, Em and Gaia

The article came out this weekend and since then I have had some wonderful comments from women about to go through treatment or empathizing with what I have been through. That's exactly what Breast Cancer Awareness hoped for from the article. I am thrilled with it – although of course shocked to see how podgy I look in the photograph.

I also was lucky enough to go to the closing night of the London Film Festival with my family and there are some lovely photos of that too. I even braved the bald head – its first outing in the film industry with former colleagues. I felt quite empowered – mostly because everyone was so kind and supportive but also because of the article and the love I have been shown not only by my friends and family but by strangers as well.

The film was *Saving Mr. Banks* starring Emma and Tom Hanks – a lovely film about the cantankerous writer of Mary Poppins and Walt Disney, who spent almost twenty years wooing her so that he could make the movie. I highly recommend it – both Em and Tom Hanks are superlative in it.

The next highlight for me will be surgery on Thursday – I will be two-thirds of the way through treatment once that is done (unless they find other naughty things when they biopsy the nodes or the breast tissue). I was rereading the early postings on this blog and pretty much everything that the oncology team had warned me about has come to pass. I have had all the side effects – especially peeved about the bloating. I honestly thought that I would come through this cancer thinner. Very cross-making as I have put on over five kilos since chemo started. In old money that's a stone in weight. Hopefully, once I am through surgery and on my health regime, that will fall off. Here's hoping.

I will post surgery results probably after the weekend. I have 100 per cent confidence in my surgery team so I am not nervous at all. My surgeon is renowned for something called 'the flick' which is an incision around the areola of the breast and then a little flick above it. Apparently (and from looking at photos) it is barely noticeable when healed. What will be noticeable to me will be a smaller left breast. I had Richard take some photos of it at the weekend (well, it was his birthday) but they are not for posting, just for me to have a record and a comparison.

Onwards and upwards. x

Operation preparation

23 OCTOBER 2013

I was not surprised to read that a school in Rotherham had had problems with children emulating *South Park*'s 'Kick a Ginger Day'. What with the huge hike in gas and electricity prices and the escalation of the war in Syria; America's bankruptcy; more people being trafficked today than at the height of the slave trade; the UN letting onto the Security Council some of THE worst offenders in the world with regard to human rights and violence, it is of little surprise that people are turning violent towards the only 'ethnic' minority not covered by race discrimination legislation – the redheads. Typical.

For those of you who want to participate there is a website called www.kickagingerday.com which has useful tips on how to spot ginger and differentiate between real and dyed red hair and why you shouldn't kick a redhead as they have souls but real gingers are fair game. They also dispel the myth that there is a rumoured 'Hug a Ginger Day'. For those of you interested I think I fell into the category of redhead rather than ginger by their definition and please don't kick me as I have quite enough to deal with right now.

I of course don't yet have enough hair to know whether it will come back as ginger/Titian/red/flame/whatever you want to call it. Backlit I do look a little like a fluffy boiled egg and as far as I can see it appears white at the front (and very patchy) and darker at the sides – so I am clearly either getting a Mallen streak style (1970s TV adaptation of a Catherine Cookson novel), or a comb over in silver grey.

I have now signed all the consent forms for my surgery on Thursday and have to turn up at the hospital at 8 a.m. to have a wire inserted into my breast (not so someone can eavesdrop on the surgeons) so that they can find the right spot. Apparently the tumour has shrunk so much that they can no longer feel it by hand. Either that or my dense breasts have hidden it, like so many other things.

By Thursday evening I will be lopsided in the façade but hopefully cancer-cell free. They will also remove the nodes under my arm (axillary) and I will have a drain there. Once I can lift that arm over my head they will discharge me. These days the worst place for sick people to be is in hospital so I should be home (with drain) on Friday evening or Saturday morning. I am told that the drain is not like something Rentokil have to deal with but is discreet, almost like carrying a bottle of water, and will even fit into a handbag. Not sure that's how I will carry it around. If it is anything like the other stuff I carry around in my sack-like handbags it will spill, get bits of tissue stuck to it and end up with a sticky lipgloss coating. I will need to rethink the portability of the drain.

Any practical suggestions welcome.

Operation

26 OCTOBER 2013

This is just a very quick post to say everything went well and I was discharged from hospital only twelve hours after I got onto the ward after surgery. I am at home being looked after by Esther and Em. I have a tube from under my armpit into a drain (bottle). I have a neat scar around my nipple with a little flick off to the left. They will biopsy the tissue and we will have results in ten days.

Operation and post-operation

28 OCTOBER 2013

We checked into the hospital at 7 a.m. Almost immediately I was seen by the surgeon Ms G – who was very chirpy and informative. Clearly this is the bit she loves – being in control of the knife.

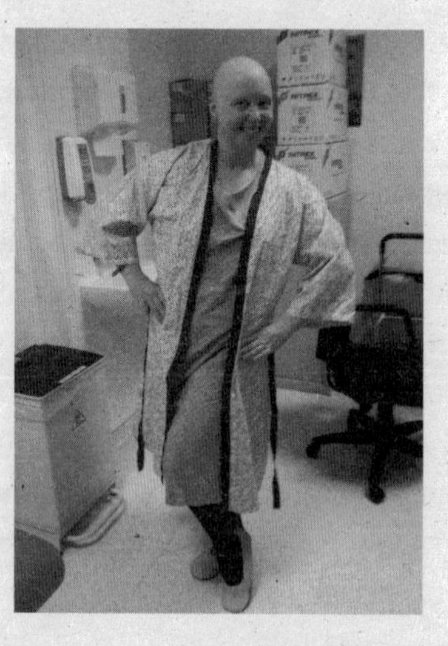

Modelling hospital gown (covered in 'property of hospital'), support socks and foam slippers. Eat your heart out, Gisele

She drew an arrow pointing down to my left breast – I felt like an Amazon package with a 'This way up' sticker. I could've done with a 'Fragile, handle with care' one as well.

She pootled off with her acolytes in tow and my next meeting was with the anaesthetist – Dr Dreamy. He was so beautiful I wondered if he was an actor brought in for the day. The nurses had warned me that Dr D was scrumptious but he was disarmingly handsome and charming. I felt crushed. No hair (a given), no make-up (upon request) and the ensemble provided by the hospital did nothing for my self-esteem. It was further crushed to smithereens when he asked me if I was 'nil by mouth'. The letter I had received said I could have breakfast at 5.30 a.m and being the dutiful patient I had done so…Oh dear, surgery would have to be delayed until after 12 noon. I couldn't bear that I had let down Dr Dreamy. I felt like I was back at school and a teacher had given me that 'I am so disappointed in you' look when your homework came back covered in red marks.

Luckily there was a pre-surgery procedure that had to be done which filled in some of the time. We trundled off to the Cancer Centre for me to have a wire inserted into the breast. Quite literally about a foot of thin wire. The sort you use for hanging pictures. Apparently the tumour had shrunk so much that they needed a guiding wire for the surgery. It was uncomfortable as it was done using an ultrasound machine – more indelible black markings put on the boob to guide the surgeons (getting a little worried now that they need pen marks to know where to cut) and then the wired boob went into the mammogram machine for more pictures – ouch and ouch.

My team from the Cancer Centre all popped by to wish me luck and give me hugs, etc. I do feel that I am part of a team – only at this point one of them could've offered to have surgery to spare me.

We returned to the surgical reception and had to wait for five hours – umm. Not great. Lots of other people also waiting. No great mags to read and pretty hard chairs to sit on – perhaps this was to prep me for further discomfort.

At 1 p.m. I was collected to go to theatre. You walk there yourself and I was met in the theatre reception by Dr Dreamy who had got over his huff about my early-morning breakfast. He really is far too good-looking and nice. He had two students with him learning the ropes – both women and both blushed every time he addressed them. I doubt either will learn anything under him (as it were) as they would be too distracted. Dr Dreamy lives near me and his wife was an actress on *Holby City* for years – he had had to give her doctoring tips (you can give me tips any time, Dr Dreamy). They were very efficient at putting in the drips and then putting me to sleep.

Three hours later I woke up in recovery – what a nice and jolly lot the nurses are. That may have been the general anaesthetic talking, of course. Ms G popped by very pleased with her handiwork. 'Have you had a look?' she said – I felt mean as of course I hadn't looked, partly because I was hooked up to oxygen and drips but also because I am a wimp and am squeamish about wounds. I lied of course, so as I wouldn't hurt her feelings. She was very pleased. She has even given me her famous 'flick'. And luckily she was able to save the nipple. Hurrah.

Then Dr Dreamy popped by and I gushed about how wonderful his anaesthetic was . . . I am such a creep. What seemed like moments later but was in fact a couple of hours they offered to let Esther and Em come and see me. Poor Esther had been in the hospital since 7 a.m. and it was now almost 7 p.m. All the nurses went into a twitter when Em appeared and Dr Dreamy got completely star-struck and blushed a lot. Ha. That made me feel better. When Em went off to get her bag he rushed up to me babbling. 'Am I doing OK? I'm not coming over as an idiot, am I?' he said. No, I reassured him and for a moment felt a little smug as I was now in control.

That moment passed quickly when I had to pee and Em had to come with me . . . you know you are sick when your nearest and dearest have to help you to the toilet.

I was then taken to the acute/short stay ward and various tests, etc., were done and I was given oxygen and morphine – hurrah, finally a class A drug. Em went off to forage for food and then I sent her home. The evening shift came on (a very lovely Ugandan nurse in charge with Filipino nursing assistants). They were all very jolly and my bed was by their station so I didn't sleep but managed to con them out of more oral morphine at around 2 a.m.

By 6 a.m. we were woken up and our vitals checked and I got up. The whole ward was in a tizz as the consultants were due on their rounds. Ms G, who is always eccentrically dressed, arrived looking quite sartorially elegant apart from her shoes which were an odd colour – like a blood orange with a large purple bow on them. They really brought out her green eyeshadow. But as Greg reminded me, she was hired for her ability as a surgeon not as a fashion guru. And anyway, I couldn't talk as I was wearing a hospital gown. I had hastily (and in the dark) put on some make-up just in case Dr Dreamy was visiting. On reflection it might have been better to wait for some light before slapping on eye make-up. I looked like a cross between Johnny Depp as Tonto and, well, Johnny Depp in *Pirates*.

Ms G had her acolytes with her and everyone stood back to admire her handiwork – after a bit of prodding she pronounced me ready to go home and it was only just 7.30 a.m. I had been on the ward twelve hours.

After Ms G had left Dr Dreamy appeared, looking even more gorgeous in the early-morning light. I hope he felt the same about me and didn't comment on my strange make-up as he is a gentleman, of course.

It then took four hours until the pharmacist dispensed going-home drugs (not allowed oral morphine but have been given something called tramadol – henceforth known as trampoline – only to be taken in extremis as it is as strong as morphine and some people have been known to talk to dead relatives on it). I was dispatched homewards with a sore boob, a tube sticking out from my armpit and a bottle on the end of it filled with . . . I leave that to the imagination. This is the drain that I have to keep in for ten days and which we have to measure the fluid every day and report to the hospital. It's very weird to have something attached to you and occasionally I forget and get up only to have it clatter to the floor. Luckily it is sealed.

The pre-op letter had said I would need a support bra and Esther didn't feel my Rigby and Peller lacy jobs or my Agent Provocateur were suitable candidates so she went off to buy me a sports bra. I guess when I am better I can always take up sport. (Is that a flying pig I see?)

Since being at home I have been so well cared for by Esther and Em. Esther has even helped me shower and dress. That's really testing a friendship. I have been inundated with flowers and visits and messages.

Sadly, I haven't been talking to dead relatives whilst on the tramadol but have enjoyed some wild dreams – too wild to mention on a family blog.

We see the surgeon next Tuesday when hopefully the drain will have also come out. For now I have it wrapped in a piece of silk around my waist. Well, it had to be silk – can't let our standards slip now, can we? Even in recovery from surgery.

Poverty and breast cancer

30 OCTOBER 2013

There was a remarkable report published this week linking breast cancer deaths to poverty. Remarkable because it seems to me that cancer is the great leveller. It hits people regardless of background, postcode or class. But the University of Cambridge has researched women diagnosed with breast cancer between 2006 and 2010 and has found that women from poorer backgrounds are diagnosed at a later stage than women from affluent areas. They seem to think that poorer women don't want to bother their GPs with first signs of symptoms.

This seems extraordinary to me and so I have contacted the lovely Estée Lauder BCA people to see if we can't work together to tackle this. I would love to do something practical to raise awareness and if I could be an ambassador for early detection I would feel that this period of my life hasn't been a complete waste. Perhaps they could send me off to talk to women in more impoverished areas of the UK. I think I could connect with women regardless of background – after all, I am not a native Londoner and come from modest northern roots. My mother was an immigrant (from Hungary) and with having Tindy in my life I have a little understanding of immigration and the very particular problems associated with that.

I will keep you posted and when I work out the technology I will post the link to the news report on the study.

I got this from my father's cousin in America in response to this posting:

Hello Darling Clare,

I just read your blog mentioning the report on the correlation between breast cancer and poverty. We have the same link here in the US but possibly for different basic reasons. The majority of working poor women here have not had any access to health care other than the Emergency Room at their local hospital. It is crazy that in the richest nation in the world, a large percentage of women never see a doctor unless they are often too sick to gain any value from 'preventive' practices. In addition, once they are diagnosed with breast cancer it becomes a 'pre-existing condition' which means that no health insurance company will take them.

The indigent have a coverage called 'Medicaid' which is pretty good – if they have the means to access it. America relies very heavily on car transportation which most of the indigent do not have.

Time is also a problem since working poor women here lose pay if they don't show up at work and most doctors work Monday through Friday 8–5 which cuts into most low-paying job schedules.

One of the major causes of bankruptcy in the US is huge medical bills – and if those bills arise from any form of cancer they can run into the hundreds of thousands of dollars.

The new Affordable Care Act will solve many of these problems since it does away with the 'pre-existing condition' clause and allows the working poor to buy inexpensive health care. Known as 'Obamacare' our conservative party is pathologically opposed to this law and is doing everything it can to obstruct its implementation.

However, in Britain where you have universal health care, none of these reasons – apart from possibly the scheduling problem– should be the reason for poor women failing to seek health care for themselves. It would be interesting to see what the other reasons are. I know that at least for some in the US, language is a huge barrier for our poor women to seek help. Here in Florida we have a population that speaks seventy-two different languages, and that stops women especially going to the doctor unless she is sure she is not going to have a language problem. If she has children, many times she will have to take an older child with her to the doctor to act as interpreter. I have no knowledge if similar conditions exist in the UK.

I applaud your willingness to tackle this problem and will be interested in hearing about your experiences on that journey.

I feel that Jane is right. We are so lucky to have a National Health Service and this should mean that we all have an equal opportunity to health care... In reality, this country is divided along economic and geographic lines and as I keep saying I have been fortunate in the postcode lottery. I can't tackle the woeful inadequacies of the NHS in some parts of the country but I do feel strongly that I can help women from whatever background to be aware of this disease. Any thoughts welcome.

Results

31 OCTOBER 2013

I am seeing the oncologist today at 4 p.m. to learn the results of the tissue biopsies removed at surgery. I still have the drain in my armpit which is a pain both literally and figuratively. I will post results later but I am very positive about the outcome. I can't believe that the double whammy of chemo and surgery won't have worked and I still have radiotherapy to go.

Results and buckets

1 NOVEMBER 2013

I saw the onco-plastic surgeon today. Good news is that she thinks she caught all the cancer. When she was in the breast she found another cancer tumour also Grade 3 like the original tumour. She cut around both and the cells surrounding the tumours were cancer free. Of the fifteen lymph nodes she removed (all the ones under my left armpit), three of them had cancer. Phew, she feels very confident they got everything.

I start radiotherapy probably the week after my birthday, so third week in November, and that will go on for four to six weeks. I will meet the radiotherapy team next week and will report back.

They took out the drain from the armpit but I am leaking. Apparently the fluid is called seroma and will keep leaking out until the hole is closed or it will form large bumps which will have to be aspirated every few days. Hmmm.

But aside from the news from the surgeon I have other news. We are going to Iceland on Thursday to see the Northern Lights. It is on the bucket list. This list doesn't necessarily mean you are going to die although the name comes from 'kicking the bucket', i.e. dying – apparently, when someone was hanged they kicked the bucket away at death.

Anyway, I don't yet know all the science but NASA says that this year and most of the next one are the best years for fifteen years to see the aurora borealis. It is something to do with solar winds. We have been following the NASA website for months and this weekend makes sense for our itineraries – if it's a full moon then you can't see the lights. I will report back both with the science and other great facts.

For now I am cancer free, hurrah.

xxx

Deciduous nails

14 NOVEMBER 2013

Chemo really is the gift that keeps on giving… now my nails are dropping off. They had gone this horrid white/yellow/grey colour which I had artfully disguised with some Clinique nail polish for sensitive nails sent to me by Estée Lauder when I started having problems, but instead of nail varnish I clearly need ship's varnish. So far I have lost a thumbnail and a middle fingernail. It's fine if I avoid anything dangerous like tying my shoelaces, opening a package or doing up buttons/zips… which basically confines me to a onesie and mittens.

I saw the radiotherapy team yesterday. I will need four weeks' radio which should start in the next ten days. I will have to go in for a pre-meet where they will find the most uncomfortable position for me to lie in, completely still, for ten minutes on one side and ten on the other. There will be two points of entry – my neck and my breast. They will also give me two (permanent) tattoos so that they can accurately position the X-ray beam. So not only have I had a nipple piercing during cancer but now I am getting a tattoo. I feel very radical. Greg thinks I should get a cartoonist friend of ours to come up with a funky way of joining the two tattoos – not the run-of-the-mill Maori or runes for me... perhaps a 'This way up' sign?

I hope that this will mean that it will all be over by Christmas but, as Greg ruefully pointed out, that was what was said in Verdun in September 1914...Very helpful.

On the hair front I have about as much hair as a three-month-old baby. Rather alarmingly, I seem to be getting sideburns. I don't remember having those before so this could be yet another gift of chemo. Perhaps I will say I grew them for 'Movember' (just as October was Breast Cancer Awareness, November is Prostate Cancer Awareness and men are encouraged to grown moustaches for money). Esther thinks they may fall out or perhaps I can get a job in a circus if they don't.

I will update the blog with our Iceland adventure later, but yes, we saw the Northern Lights (another tick off my bucket list) and ate puffin... not a whole one, mind you. That would be wrong or possibly wronger.

Birthday joy

19 NOVEMBER 2013

It's my birthday today and I enter my fiftieth year cancer free. Hurrah. I start the radiotherapy journey this week with the tattoos and a CT scan. The actual radiotherapy will start in a few weeks and will sadly go on through Christmas and into the New Year but then it will all be over.

I will post the Iceland blog and pictures ASAP. Tonight I am off to see Dame Edna's farewell tour and we will have champers with her after the show, so an excellent start to my half-century year.

Thank you for all your lovely birthday messages and responses on the blog. I feel very lucky despite the cancer thingy.

xxx

The tattooed woman

26 NOVEMBER 2013

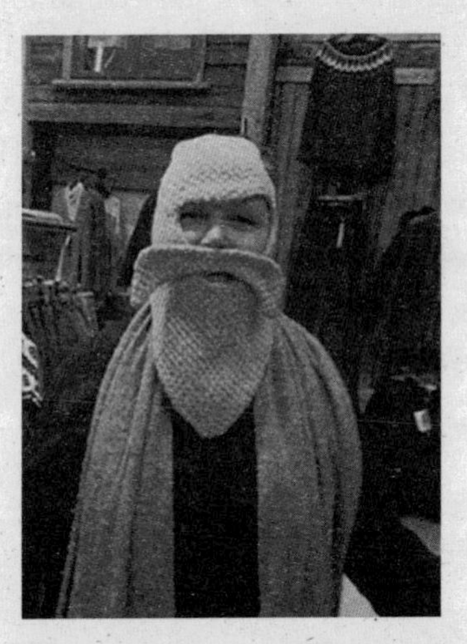

Icelandic headgear for the follically challenged

I went for my pre-radiotherapy assessment last Friday. It was in the basement of the main hospital – two floors underground – great big thick walls of lead and large humming machines. My first test was to see if I could lie 'comfortably' on the 'bed' under the CT radiation machine. Hmmm. It is like lying on a photocopier. Clearly, I am going to have to practise at my local copy shop. Quite literally, you lie on a metal and glass top. There is a metal triangular wedge for your knees and head. I am expected to lie still for forty-five minutes. Really??? I thought the mammogram machine was ludicrous – all hard edges – but this takes the prize.

To make me more comfortable they gave me a softer headrest. Texturally, it is like one of those Oasis things you use for flower arranging. So less hard than metal but hardly soft. I had to raise my arms above my head to hang onto a bar above. Ouch.

Then the two nurses got out metal rulers and something resembling a pair of compasses and a sextant-like object. None of which would have been out of place on *Master and Commander* but seemed odd in a radiotherapy suite.

They attached metal wire under and around my breasts – using Sellotape to keep it in place. Then they drew on me with a variety of felt pens and got out the metal rulers and measured distances between the breasts and sides of the machine. Then they covered me with dots, switched on a green cross hair and readjusted me, the dots and the wire bra. Once they were satisfied they shunted me into the machine – a large doughnut with a revolving metal core... all very *Goldfinger* I thought as I lay there.

'You expect me to talk?'

'No, Mr Bond, I expect you to die.'

Thereafter they pressed buttons and I went in and out of the machine a couple of times. They readjusted the measurements – a whole new set and colour of felt tips used and they pronounced themselves satisfied. They asked me to lie still, take shallow breaths and relax…of course, it's very easy to do all of that when you are not strapped onto a moving photocopier covered in wire and ballpoint join-the-dots. Hmm. Then they went out of the room and the machine whirred into life. I still can't get used to these machines. It is like being in the engine room of the *Starship Enterprise* with Scotty pushing the dilithium crystals to the max, Cap'n. All very odd.

After a few minutes the nurses returned and untaped the wire and this time made permanent tattoo marks on me – one either side of either breast – one in the middle of my sternum and one above my left breast. These are their markers for the cross hairs of the machine.

So that's that.

I start for real on 12 December and will go in every day bar weekends and will be allowed Christmas Day, Boxing Day and New Year's Day off but will have to go in on two Saturdays to make up for the holiday.

I have been accepted on a clinical trial so instead of twenty days' radiation I will only have fifteen days' as some of those days I will have a boost in radiation. Joy. I am happy that it will be fifteen days and the whole thing will be done by the end of the first week in January.

Now I have to practise lying on a photocopier with my arms over my head for at least forty-five minutes. How hard can that be?

On a sad note... Esther leaves tomorrow. She has been here for almost five months and I suppose it is reasonable that she wants her life back. I have tried hiding her passport but she has taken to carrying it with her just in case. I won't embarrass her too much at this stage but all I can say is, THANK YOU. She has been amazing and wonderful and everyone should be lucky enough to have an Esther in their lives. I couldn't have managed without her and it is remarkable that she hasn't wanted to kill me. I would have killed me.

And now an update on the hair front. When I was having chemo and had lost all of my hair, all my body hair in particular, I couldn't get goosebumps. Now my whole body is covered in goosebumps as the hair follicles are once again in demand. It's a very strange feeling to be bumpy. I seem to be getting a lot of extra down – I feel as though I am growing my own onesie in time for winter. I don't remember being that hairy or downy. Perhaps this is another lovely cancer gift. The beard and sideburns are progressing well. The hair on my head is about 2 millimetres long and is coming through in a variety of colours. I used shampoo for the first time in five months. It's a little early to get excited about hair products but a girl can try.

I promised to post a blog about Iceland and will do so shortly.

But for now, goodbye from the tattooed bearded woman. x

Medicinema

27 NOVEMBER 2013

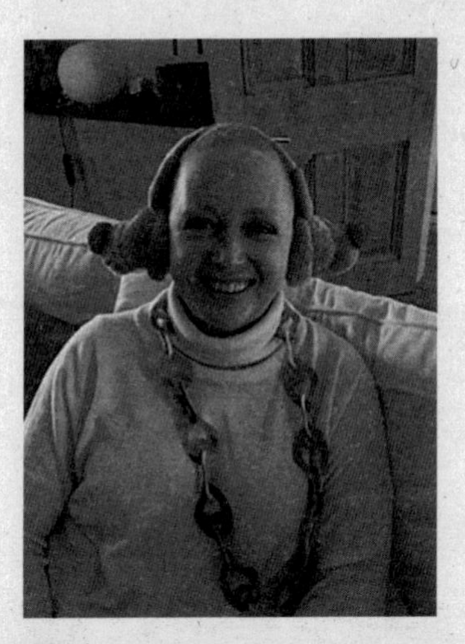

New headgear for Christmas

Last week we threw a film premiere for the lovely staff at the Macmillan Cancer Centre and over two hundred of them turned up. Medicinema organized it for me. They are a wonderful charity that I would love to work with when I am through all my treatment. Do look at their website at www.medicinema.org.uk.

At the screening I thanked all the staff, without whom I would have hair, nails, a sense of taste, but I would also have cancer. All joking aside, the staff are what make the hospital and I have been very lucky. I still want to try and find a way of helping women less fortunate than me and will be proposing a scheme to Breast Cancer Awareness when I am out the other side of treatment.

On the hair front – I have a Number 1 crew cut. I now look less like a cancer victim and more like an angry National Front yob. I am still growing facial hair and eyelashes (at last, hurrah) but am rather poor on other hair fronts, as it were. Who knew that hair grows at such different rates?

Radiotherapy starts next week so for now I am building myself up by practising lying on as many uncomfortable surfaces as possible – I am practically planking. If you don't know what it is check out this website www.planking.me.

Happy festive season.

Savvy aunty

1 DECEMBER 2013

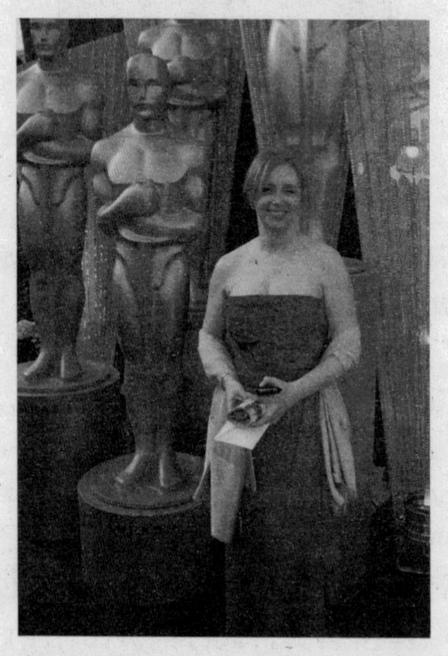

In the old days when I had hair and a job... posing here with a lot of bald bronzed hunks

I learned a new acronym last night: PANK – Professional Aunty No Kids. It seems that there are a lot of us. In the past we would have been called Maiden Aunts: MANKs – Maiden Aunt No Kids. Now we are seen as cool, perhaps because we can afford to buy cool presents and treats. I am an aunty to my niece and nephew who call me Aunty Bobs. I have two godchildren in India who call me Clare Aunty and a goddaughter in Chichester who calls me Aunty Bear. Whatever the term I feel very auntvuncular??? If an uncle is avuncular what is an aunty?

I think I am more of a SPANK: Semi-Professional Aunt No Kids or perhaps a BLANK: Based London Aunty No Kids or maybe a (dare I say it) W-ANK: Worldwide Aunty No Kids or even a SANK: Single Aunty No Kids, or even a RANK: Riotous Aunty No Kids. This could go on for ever…

My niece says I am 'out of control': OOCANK?

I realized that acronyms have crept into everyday life and even into my cancer. It is a DCIS, ER8, PR7, HER2 negative. I am told that the nurses also write acronyms or coded phrases on charts to describe the patient. ONGAR means one stop short of barking (mad). This is because Ongar is the penultimate stop on the Tube line that goes to Barking. What, I wonder, does mine say? I hope smiley, nice, cheerful and positive but who knows?

I saw my breast cancer nurse this week as I am still not sure about tamoxifen. The numerical stats on it preventing breast cancer are not overwhelmingly positive and the side effects are horrible and legion. I have had enough of side effects. As I write yet another nail has fallen off and my joints are aching – possibly because the bone marrow is expelling the chemo. I still am growing hair – annoyingly still in the wrong places.

I asked my nurse about trying to control the cancer through diet and lifestyle changes. I produce too much oestrogen which in the pre-cancerous cells can lead them to go rogue. The tamoxifen is an oestrogen inhibitor. Short of growing a set of balls it seems that it is hard to control my propensity to produce this hormone. She agreed to look into a different drug for me. They took more blood and will let me know my hormone levels and whether I can start with something different.

I start radiotherapy this week. An actress who lives nearby (not a relative, I hasten to add) asked me how I was. When she heard I was starting three weeks of radio she said, 'Oh, how lovely, I much prefer doing radio to TV.'

Quality Assurance

6 DECEMBER 2013

My radiotherapy was postponed as apparently I had failed 'quality assurance' tests... I have no idea what that means. I suspect that the pre-planning data was somehow incorrectly processed. So I don't start radiotherapy now until Monday.

Trust me, eh?!

x

Irradiate

16 DECEMBER 2013

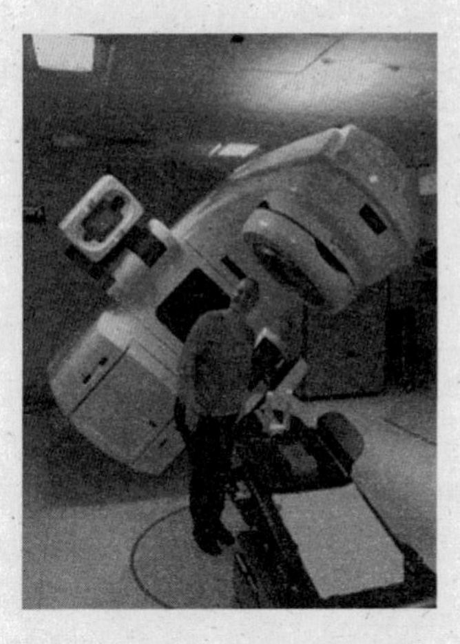

No kidding – it was like walking onto the bridge of the Starship *Enterprise*, albeit art direction by the NHS. A long windy lead-lined corridor in the bowels and basement of the hospital led to this machine. This photo gives an idea of scale and also you can see the photocopier bed I have to lie on.

First the radiologists moved me into position on the photocopier and kneaded my fat and podge into the right position – guided by the tattoos and also green intersecting laser lights. They also drew on me (just for fun) and measured me with metal rulers and callipers. I really did feel like a ball of dough.

They then explained that the machine would move round me into three different positions as I am being irradiated through my neck area, side of breast and breast bone. The room is cold because 'the machine likes it to be cold'. As Steph said, it was all a little

Terminator-like the way they referred reverentially to the machine. Perhaps even a bit HAL-like.

After they had kneaded me into place (with my arms above my head gripping onto two bars) they asked me to lie still for around thirty mins. They then scurried out of the room, hit an alarm bell to warn others about the radiation and I lay there, trying to imagine myself on a beautiful beach or lovely hotel room or anywhere but the basement of the hospital.

There's something very disconcerting about people scurrying away after hitting an alarm and leaving you with a machine that seems to growl and groan as it moves around you. It hummed and buzzed and the bed shook slightly as it moved me into proximity to the machine.

It did almost feel like it was awake and watching me. The top of it – which looks a little like an overweight *Star Wars* Stormtrooper – had what felt like an electronic eye above me which whirred and blinked and I guess that was what was handing out the radiation as it moved into three different positions. Having watched a lot of *Walking with Dinosaurs* I have decided to call the machine radiosaurus. It did sort of look at me in a knowing inquisitive way, as though it were sizing me up to eat. I couldn't help anthropomorphizing it... just to make it seem less metal.

The lovely technicians popped in a few times as the first part of the procedure was them taking images of the areas to be treated.

The actual irradiation only took about fifteen minutes but the photos and preparation was around thirty minutes. From door to door it was three hours. That's every day bar Christmas Day and

Boxing Day and New Year's Day. I get this Saturday and Sunday off but next week I will have to go in on Saturday as well. Joy.

I did lie there and think of Marie Curie, killed by radiation of course, but also about her astounding contribution to this process and medical science. Unlike chemo this treatment is topical – i.e. it goes right into the cells where the cancer was and perhaps still is. Although the surgeons are confident they got rid of the two tumours, they can't catch every pre-cancerous cell so radiation kills them off. Here's to the death rays of radiation.

Happy Christmas

25 DECEMBER 2013

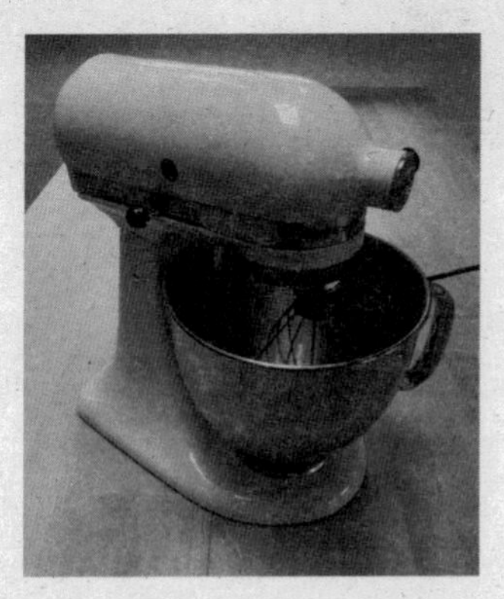

Spot the difference – this is a food mixer but doesn't it bear a resemblance to the radiosaurus machine?

I am on Day 7 of 15 in radiotherapy. As I understand it (and I am not a physics major) I am being shot through with targeted proton beams. It still all sounds very *Star Trek* to me.

Happy radioactive Christmas x

Lie nice and still

30 DECEMBER 2013

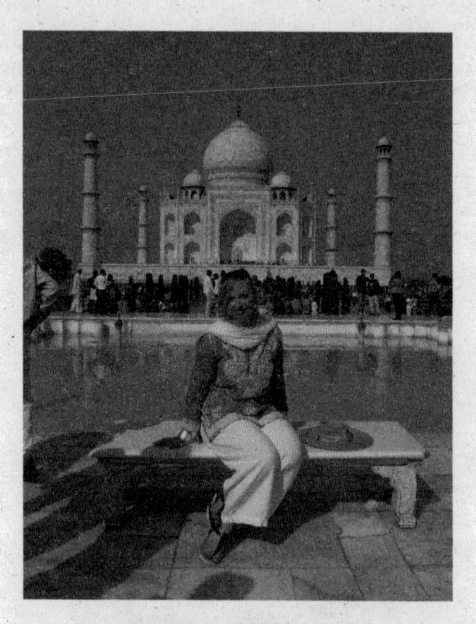

Quite like Diana at the Taj

Every time the radiographers rush out of the room they say to me, 'Lie nice and still.' I am not sure I can lie 'nice'. I can lie 'still', although it's a gargantuan effort when you are uncomfortable and cold and lying on a photocopier, with your head on an Oasis and your bum on a metal triangle. But I do try. The worst is getting an itch. I have tried that mental practice of imagining it somewhere else but that really doesn't help as I can't scratch anywhere.

The definition of 'nice', according to the *Oxford Dictionary*, means 'giving pleasure or satisfaction: pleasant or attractive' or when used about a person it means 'good-natured or kind'. It can be used ironically, for example 'not unpleasant' or it can be used to mean ‘fastidious or scrupulous’. I am not sure that any of those covers lying nicely. Perhaps it means satisfactorily. Its origins are Middle English, apparently, and it meant ‘stupid’ from Old French, and in Latin ‘*nescius*’ means ignorant or not knowing. I can certainly lie there being stupid and ignorant (especially about the radiation being used).

It was also used in medieval times to mean coy or reserved. And I am not able to be either of those when lying there. As soon as I get into the lead-lined room I have to take my top off and lie still so that the radiographers can join up my tattoos with pen marks and then measure distance with rulers and a calibrated light from the radiosaurus. Any chance of being coy is taken away completely, although they do put a sheet of kitchen roll over my tits before running out of the room. So perhaps I am lying there coyly.

In the Taj Mahal in Agra – one of the architectural wonders of the world and visited by millions every year – there is a sign in the inner sanctum, where the sarcophagus of Shah Jahan and his wife lies, that says, ‘Be Quite.’ In all the years that I have been visiting India no one has pointed out the spelling mistake. So I guess if I can be ‘quite’ in the Taj, I can lie ‘nice’ in the University College Hospital.

Today is New Year’s Eve and I will have completed ten of my fifteen radio sessions. Hurrah. I am almost finished with cancer treatments and can start 2014 free from this disease. It also means I have to get my life and my body back. Both daunting prospects. So no New Year resolutions for me but lots of post-cancer ones.

If you’re celebrating tomorrow, party nice and be quite in 2014.

x

Side effects

31 DECEMBER 2013

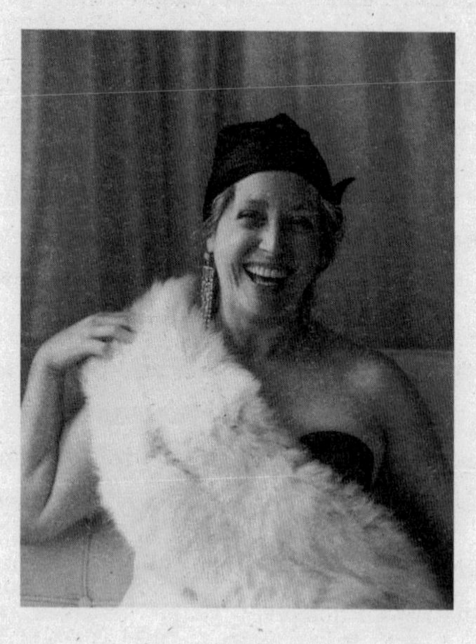

One thing I won't miss AT ALL are side effects. I'm not sure why they aren't called 'front effects'... I think all the effects of chemo and radio are full-frontal not side issues. They are a misnomer.

The side effects of radiotherapy are burning skin (check), nausea (check), upset tummy (check) and extreme fatigue (triple check). On top of that I have such aching useless limbs. It's like having the flu.

My lovely radiographer tells me that's all normal and that it will take a month before they can scan me and check the cells have been nuked as right now they are all in distress. I know how they feel.

I had to see a chiropodist today as my toenails and feet suffered horribly with chemo. She was lovely but told me that it would be years before they return to normal. She did make me laugh, though, when I asked about working during the holidays, she said it was fine as they were 'having it off' now until Tuesday. I wish!

My New Year's resolution, apart from getting over the last cancer treatment, is to lose the chemo weight. I have six weeks until the BAFTAs – by then I need my hair to look as though it was meant to be and I want to fit into a lovely dress I bought years ago when I went to the Oscars. I've put on a stone and a half since chemo – ten kilos. Yikes. I don't think I can lose that before 17 February but I will try.

If you see me eating carbs or lazing around, please encourage me to meet my goal.

After that all I have to do is get a life . . . I don't know if you know, but I was made redundant some time ago and since May cancer has taken over my life. Now that I am about to be free of it I need to concentrate on a new career. I loved my old life but clearly it didn't agree with me healthwise. Any suggestions would be very welcome. I have lost my self-confidence through not working and aside from needing to earn money I also need to retake my place in society . . . or rather, the working world.

I do want to continue trying to find a way to increase breast cancer awareness and will cook up a plan to do that. I have been so lucky to have the treatment I have had and to have the friends I have. I am humbled every day that I am in the hospital seeing people so much less fortunate than I am. Although I don't recommend anyone going through this, it has been an amazing time. The NHS staff that I have met are so wonderful in the face of constant criticism in the press. The other patients are so courageous and the doctors and nurses are without doubt heroes and heroines.

So many people have remarked about my battle with cancer – it really isn't a battle. I gave my body over to medical science on 6 May and will get it back on 8 January. I am not brave. I just get through each day and that would be so much harder were it not for my amazing family and friends. Esther would never admit how extraordinary it was for her to give up five months of her life to look after me. But it really is an extraordinary thing. I can't ever repay that, nor do I think of her sacrifice in those terms. I think the only way I can repay that and all the other fantastic acts of kindness shown to me is that I fight for cancer awareness and do my utmost to make sure that other people are as lucky as I have been.

Sorry for the reflective nature of this blog but I am almost at the end of the road and, although I only want to look ahead with great positivity, I also need to reflect on what just happened. Please, please, tell any women you know to take care of their breasts and if they have the slightest doubt to insist on seeing a doctor. Similarly, all men need to check their testicles and not be embarrassed.

The head nurse in the Cancer Centre was telling me that only a few years ago they treated ninety women and last year that number was a hundred and seventy. If it's true and soon one in two of us will get cancer, I hope that I am your one and that you will never have to go through this.

x

Today

7 JANUARY 2014

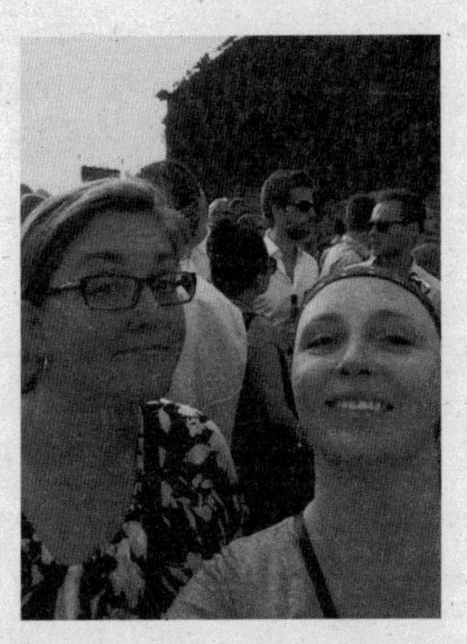

Sorry, Est, but I had to post one photo of you – this is at the Rolling Stones back in July

Today is my last day of cancer treatment. Apart from some follow-up scans and appointments I am done. It's exactly eight months (and a day) that I was diagnosed.

I can't thank you all for the support and love that you have all given me. But I have some very special thanks: to my wonderful family whose love and support has been beyond that expected from the familial nexus.

Thank you to my niece for being so strong and positive and for not worrying about me and always being 100 per cent sure that I would be fine. You are an amazing person and I love watching you grow up to be a strong independently minded woman.

Thank you to my nephew for being yourself. You make me howl with laughter and your booming, infectious laugh makes everyone smile. Thank you for your love and compassion and for your digs about me being 'ancient'.

Thank you, Em, without whom chemo and those long months would have seemed interminable. Your love and strength got me through so much. We laughed a lot and your overwhelming generosity and kindness both to me and the hospital has been beyond any call of duty.

Thank you, Greg – for being my brother and best friend. I can't begin to imagine how tough all this was on you. Since both Mum and Dad died you have been my rock. From the first moment of diagnosis to the last trip today you have seen me through all of this with such composure and love. Thank you for coming to all of the radiotherapy sessions with me – even though it is tedious and monotonous.

Thank you, Esther. You are so much part of my family even though we aren't related. Without you we would all have been so much poorer. You have been truly magnificent and your unselfishness and practical approach to this time in my life have humbled me. I know you hate being in the spotlight but live with it. I can't ever thank you enough.

Thank you, Philly, for being my inspiration. No one has handled this horrible disease as well as you. You have been through the 'wringer' and no one appreciates this more than me. It was such a comfort to me to know that everything I was going through would soon be over and that I would emerge out of it stronger.

Thank you, Emma – this was very hard on you both because of your mum and because you are so far away. Your daily calls gave me great strength and your little pep talks have helped so much – even if sometimes you had that tone of 'I am telling you this for your own good . . .' As always you were right.

Thank you, Jules – who rang every day and sent some very silly cards and whenever possible visited. You are one of the strongest women I know and the way you juggle family, job and friends is enviable.

Thank you, Fi and Richard, for all the meals on wheels, companionship and great photographs. Your positivity and practical approach have meant the world to me. Thank you for the daily phone calls and frequent visits. It couldn't have been easy when you both lead such busy lives.

Thank you to Daisy, Merv, Judith and Malcolm, and Bryan and Anna – I am so lucky to have such wonderful family support. I am in awe of Judith and Anna now that I have spent so much time in hospitals – and how you both can stay so positive and loving after days nursing ornery patients and the sick.

Thank you, Rose. This has been hard on you and even though sometimes you worry that you couldn't find the right words – with this disease there are no right words.

Thank you, Steph and Will – for your long-distance support and love. Surprising you in Miami was a goal I set myself during chemo and I think it helped me so much to aim for that. Thank you for coming and visiting and staying with me during radio. I know you love a hospital, Steph, but I don't want to be in one again for a while.

Thank you, John. Your healing spirit and great kindness to me has been such a comfort. I have grown to love Reiki and also to relax into the moment through you.

Thank you, Fen and all the Hollands and the Jamaican clans. You have been so amazing at keeping in touch and sending me your love. Thank you for offering to help me recuperate in January. You may regret it.

Thank you, Vivien, Isabel and all the Universal girls and boys for your weekly cards and messages. They made me laugh and brightened every day for me. You are an extraordinary group of talented and loving young people and I am very lucky to know you all. Thank you also to Sally and James D. and his mum for constant visits and news of the film world.

Thank you, Michael H. – your kindness in offering a change of scene at Beeleigh and your flowers and calls meant a lot to me.

Thank you to the Mumbai/Goan contigent. I am going to get well so I can come and annoy you in person.

Thank you to the Australian support network led by the Lees. I loved seeing you here and catching up on the madness there. Thanks also to Lachie and Teena.

Thank you to all the Miami partygoers – especially Grant (and for all his London support as well), Sue and Martin, the Lucases, Phaedon and Sue, and Sue Lucas's girls.

Thank you to the American supporters for lots of wonderful messages and Facebook stories: Cameron, get over here soon; Bryan, the spare bed is waiting; Pilar, let's work together soon – I miss you; Sabrina, so glad we reconnected – I miss you too.

Thanks also to Jo and Ellen – what an extraordinary year you guys have had too. None of us would have imagined that 2013 would look like it did. See you in Canada.

Thank you, Estée Lauder, for the Breast Cancer Awareness campaign. Don't think you have heard the last of me. I want to be involved and work hard with you to raise awareness. Thank you, Macmillan – in every way your support has been invaluable.

Thank you to all the blog followers – especially new friends like Tina, the other cancer sufferers who have read it, and everyone who has commented.

A HUGE THANK YOU to the staff of the Macmillan Cancer Centre – especially Shirley, Jackie, Lottie, Pamela, Dr Smith, Dr Jones, Dr Franks. Dr Gattuso, Dr Dreamy, all the first-floor nurses and receptionists, the vampirical phlebotomists, the radiographers, the Macmillan Centre Staff (Vicky and Nicola to name just two), and the wonderful radiotherapy team, especially Tash.

I am not sure what I will do now with the blog but maybe from time to time I will post the odd update. When I have sorted myself out and reached out to the breast cancer charities I might well use it to let you know what you can do to raise awareness. I am one of the very lucky ones and I don't want this to happen to any of you so PLEASE be breast aware and body aware 'cos as my old dad used to say, 'Life is not a rehearsal.' I am appalled that it has taken me fifty years to really hear that message.

Thank you, everyone, and apologies if I have left you out. You may not be in the list but you are in my heart.

Enough emotional welling-up

Clare (cancer free) x

Bloody side effects

24 JANUARY 2014

I know I have banged on about this before but I am not sure why side effects are so-called. Radiation burns your skin and your cells – hopefully nuking the rogue cells – and the side effect is a burn on your skin. Surely that is the main effect – front and centre – not some sideshow activity? Hence I have burns on my skin from radiotherapy. I have an unsightly red mark on my collarbone (or where my collarbone would be if it weren't for the rolls of fat – side effect of chemo). I have a blistering burn under my left armpit. Both are manageable effects of radiotherapy but in my humble opinion are not side effects.

The main side effect is fatigue – that old friend. Like with chemo I feel as though I have been unplugged from the mains. I simply get exhausted with the slightest effort.

Another long-term side effect of the cancer and the oestrogen inhibitor that I am on for years (called anastrozole – hereby referred to as Anastasia, like the fake Romanov princess) is osteoporosis. Brittle bones. I know this is almost inevitable with women of a certain age (euphemism for post-menopausal) but it is accelerated by my particular type of cancer. Weight-bearing exercise is the key – walking, yoga and Pilates.

So, armed with a great sense of optimism and an unreal sense of my own limitations, I decided to stride off last weekend. But in attempting to put on my walking shoes I managed to pull a muscle in my back. Ouch, ouch and more ouch. It was almost as bad as chemo. I was in agony. Greg hoovered me off to the osteopath who acupunctured me and manipulated me and almost a week later I can walk fairly normally although with the odd wince and accompanying squeal.

Is exercise bad for me? Clearly I need to stretch and take it very slowly when attempting more than a gentle furniture crawl.

On the hair front there is real progress. I will soon have a full beard and sideburns and body hair apiece. But the head is quite slow growing. I saw an advert on the side of a bus last week advertising a serum called 'Grow Gorgeous'. I couldn't resist and have been liberally smearing it all over. Apparently it is a hair serum which might account for my overall hirsute-ness (is that a word?).

A friend who has had breast reconstruction after her mastectomy has discovered that her new breast is hairy. Since the reconstruction was done years after the mastectomy the surgeons took skin from her thighs (and back and tummy and flesh from other parts . . . ouch, ouch, ouch) and of course if hair grows on your thighs it doesn't matter where it ends up the skin still grows hair. The indignity of breast cancer never stops.

I am going to treat us both to a course of electrolysis when I get a job. It seems the most fitting reward for our recovery.

Hair's to you all.

Grow Gorgeous.

Clare

Diamonds are a girl's best friend

18 FEBRUARY 2014

Life after treatment is, of course, wonderful but also strangely empty. Maybe I have a type of Stockholm Syndrome and perversely miss the constant attention of being a patient. I definitely DO NOT miss chemo and actually even though the radiographers were lovely I don't miss radiotherapy either. But I do feel a little abandoned.

To make up for this I went to the BAFTAs this weekend – accompanied by my friend Vincenzo and the rest of the family. Em was nominated as Best Actress for her stellar performance in *Saving Mr Banks*.

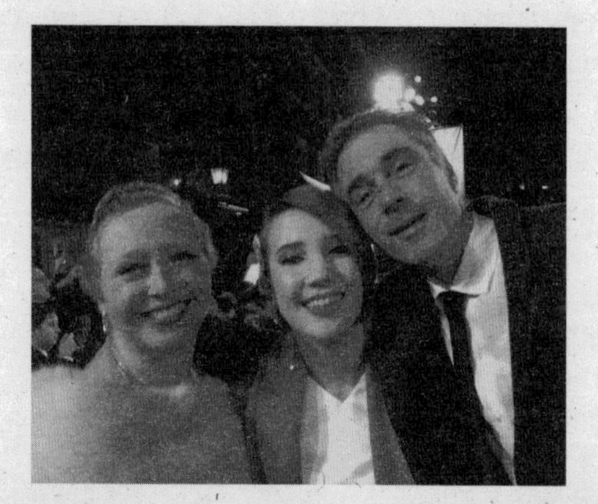

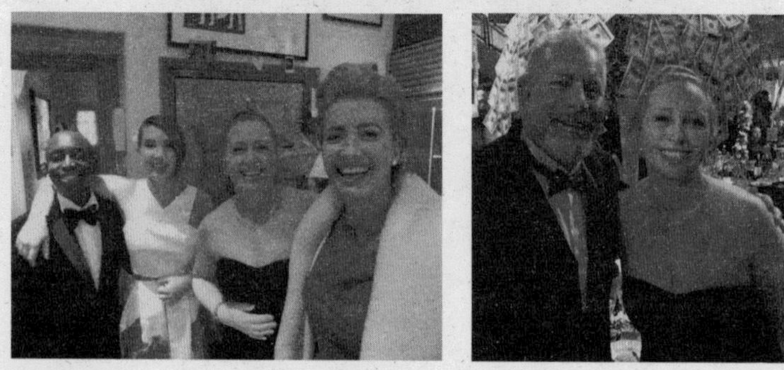

I was lent some beautiful diamonds from Boodles, a jewellery shop that has been in existence since the eighteenth century. The set was called Aurora and consisted of over sixty individual yellow, rose and white 3-carat diamonds and hundreds of smaller ones. I wore earrings, necklace and a bracelet and the whole value was around half a million pounds. They came complete with a security guard who delivered them to the house and picked them up from me at the end of the evening (2 a.m.). I felt like a princess. Ironically, everything else I was wearing (dress, fake-fur wrap and shoes) was off the high street. And as you can see I even have some hair so I wore a little beaded band in it to distract from the shortness.

People who didn't know I had cancer just thought I had gone for a radical haircut... bless them.

Gaia was dressed by Topshop and looked amazing. Tindy wore a velvet dark green smoking jacket and Greg wore a beautiful DJ. Vincenzo was in Armani and Em was in a gorgeous red dress from Maria Grachvogel.

We partied with Tom Hanks and his wife Rita, Leonardo, Christoph Waltz, Maggie Gyllenhaal and a host of other lovelies, but having had to get ready at 3 p.m. and leave by 4.30 p.m. we didn't eat until 11.30 p.m. and by 1 a.m. we were all shattered and crept home to have cheese on toast and champagne in our PJs whilst waiting for the security guard to come and take away our diamonds.

Now back to normal life. Phew.

xxx

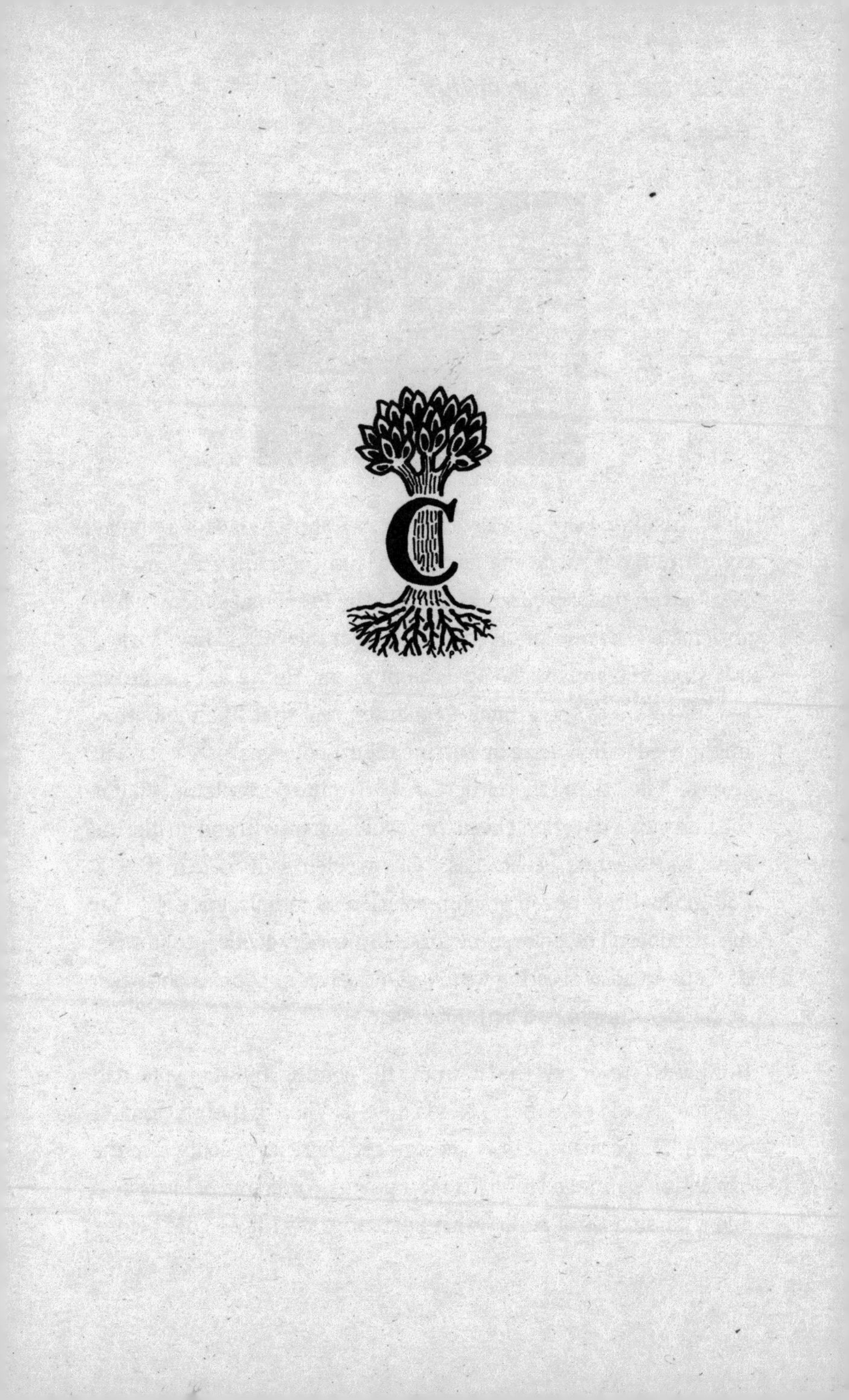

They never saw it coming

4 APRIL 2014

THE
FRENCH
ARISTOCRACY
NEVER SAW IT
COMING EITHER.
Manhattan
Mini Storage.com
STORAGE
AS LOW AS
$29
FREE
MOVE

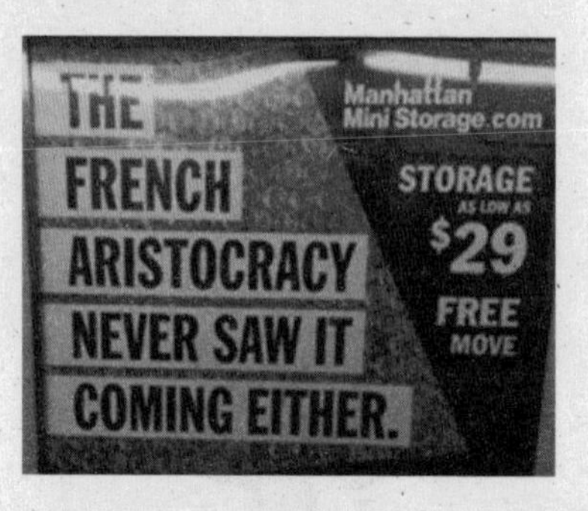

I love this sign. I saw it in New York on the subway. It's for a storage company. That made me laugh out loud (perhaps risky on the Manhattan underground) as even if the French aristocracy had anticipated the revolution I doubt whether they would have turned to a storage company to solve the problem. Here I am assuming the 'It' refers to the French Revolution and that like today they might need to downsize by putting their Louis Quatorze chairs in storage. The 'it' and the 'either' are both quite portentous. What is the message – if we don't heed the revolution we will end up like the French aristocrats, i.e. headless? Our problem sadly here in the UK and in the US is not so much revolution as complacency. And for me that doesn't mean rushing to put my worldly goods into storage. Perhaps an ad suggesting we divest ourselves of possessions when 'it' happens might be a better message.

However, I never saw the 'it' in my life coming and if anyone had told me I would get cancer I would have laughed in their faces but I wouldn't have rushed out to get storage. There is no doubt that the cancer is a watershed for me. I realize, with a mixture of bitterness and a harsh dose of reality, that I can't live my life as I did before.

Then I lived to work. Now I need to work to live and achieve this mythical work–life balance. My mother, who had a unique way of reminding me of my fallibilities, rang me one day at work and asked me what it would say on my headstone: 'She worked long hours at the office?' Harsh and, by the way, should any of you have to organize this for me I don't want a headstone and would rather go up in a firework after a brilliantly louche party.

But not yet. I am getting stronger and better every day but the lasting legacy of the cancer is impeding my progress a bit. My hair is growing and as my friend Franck said it now just looks like a bad haircut. In my more poetic moments I am sure I look like Jean Seberg in *Jules et Jim* – but in reality I look more like Paul Scholes (Man United footballer with receding ginger hairline).

My chemo brain is abating although I am still struggling for words – less the polysyllabic variety and more the ordinary everyday words of one syllable. This may, of course, be my age as well – that slow progress towards infantile speech patterns. On the physical side I am definitely improving but the new drug I am on gives me terrible joint pain and it is causing bursitis in my hips and I now have a problem with my left arm. Apparently one in twenty breast cancer sufferers gets a problem there after surgery. Mine has started off as cording, which as the name suggests means a tightening of your muscle cords. This has now morphed into something called 'adhesive capulitis' – in common parlance, a frozen shoulder.

It doesn't sound bad, does it, 'frozen shoulder'? In reality it is agony. I can't lift my left arm above the height of my ribcage and if I reach for a mug in the cupboard or my bra strap behind my shoulder the pain makes me want to vomit or faint. The worst news is that there is nothing to be done. It usually takes eighteen to twenty-four months for the condition to settle down and go away. Bloody hell. I am trying yoga and stretches but I can only do the movements lopsidedly which makes balances and warrior position a little touch and go.

Perhaps the 'it' of this ad is life after cancer. I had not anticipated feeling worse post-treatment.

I am off to get some storage and see if that solves it.

xx

Due to popular demand

22 JULY 2014

I have been asked by so many people why I haven't been blogging recently. The answer is that I really didn't have anything more to say on my cancer 'journey'... but guess what – I do.

A year to the day after my diagnosis, another close friend has been given the news that she too has breast cancer. Of my 'circle of strength' (so-called by the *Daily Mail* article) that's now three out of six of us. This is an epidemic. I can't possibly assume that I know the reason why but there is one thing that links us all – stress and impossibly stressful careers. In my case I produce too much adrenaline and cortisol and this seems to translate in my body into fibroids and clearly some of them went rogue. I also explain away my weight issues with adrenaline – blood sugar problem. Given the bad press sugar has had recently I can see the results in my body. (I don't gorge on chocolate or ice cream but I do love wine, which is where I get a lot of my sugar from.) According to the BMI scale I am clinically obese. I can give myself a little comfort in that Greg is also obese according to the scale. Those of you who know him, know that he hasn't an ounce of excess flesh on his body, but his height to weight ratio put him in that category, so clearly it is not a great way to measure obesity.

A few years ago I was travelling through Colombo airport en route from Sri Lanka. (Vincenzo and I had gone there on a SAGA holiday. I celebrated my birthday there and for the first time in a long time I felt very young, practically a teenager, when I turned forty-eight, as the average age of the group, excluding Vinne and myself, was seventy-six.) I was going to Mumbai and the planes between these troubled neighbours leave at 3 a.m. I don't know about you but I

ALWAYS look my best at 3 a.m. in strip neon airport lighting. I handed my passport over to a portly customs man who looked at the photo and then looked at me: 'You have gotten very fat,' he said. Understandably I was taken aback by this. 'That's very rude,' I said, hoping I didn't end up in a jail in Sri Lanka. 'I am just telling you how I see it,' he said. 'In your photo you look slim and now you are fat.' Jeepers. I can't even get away with it at Passport Control.

So in an effort to shift my cancer weight I have been attempting exercise. Shock horror. I was impeded by adhesive capulitis (frozen shoulder) and had a steroid injection into the muscle and can now almost do a full salute with my left arm. Philippa paid for me to have one-on-one yoga sessions with an amazing woman called Abi who is without doubt the best teacher I have ever had. She is also helping my friend recently diagnosed and now on her chemo nightmare. It is definitely helping although the steroid-enhanced left arm now makes me look like a lopsided Popeye.

Talking of amazing yoga teachers, I learned last night of the death from breast cancer of another phenomenal woman who has taught my family yoga for decades. She was a strong and extraordinary woman who was diagnosed ten years ago. She elected to treat the disease in a very different way to me. Using a combination of ground-breaking injections and homeopathy with limited surgery. For a decade she was healthy and then the bloody thing returned with a vengeance six months ago. I admired her totally for her commitment to non-traditional cancer treatment and although I would not have chosen her path we were all 100 per cent supportive. She died earlier this week at such a young age. I am immensely proud and privileged to have known her.

Since finishing in January I have been a bit at sea. Literally and figuratively. Figuratively – I went through withdrawal. I had been the centre of so much attention and activity and during radiotherapy had been in the hospital every day. Suddenly I was cut loose and told, 'See you in October.' Abandoned. No scroll or parchment to say I had passed the test or even some kind of medal. Just told to go home and get better.

My energy levels were very poor through February and March, and the hospital offered me complimentary treatments at the homeopathic hospital and counselling. They have both been marvellously helpful, especially the psychiatry. I had my first session the day my friend was diagnosed by the same team who looked after me. To say I was cross about her is an understatement – I was livid. I honestly assumed in my usual panegyric way that because I had been through cancer no one else close to me should have to go through it. I was fulfilling the statistics. Guess what – like most things in my life I was wrong. It doesn't work like that. So seeing the shrink has been very helpful and by May I was feeling rumbustious and back to my old self.

My hair is growing well and I have even had a haircut but I am still lacking in the body hair department with thin eyebrows and short stumpy eyelashes. So I can't be up to date with Cara Delevingne-style bushy eyebrows but I have rediscovered my love of fake eyelashes – or rather eyelash extensions. I have even introduced them to other friends.

And now to the literal being at sea. Sabrina, who lives in LA, quite rightly decided to celebrate her birthday with a fabulous holiday, coming to London first and then flying me out to Nice to join her and some gorgeous friends for a few days on a luxury yacht going round the Côte d'Azur and then some time in St-Tropez. It is ironic that I am completely broke and yet holiday in great style. I am so lucky to have such generous friends. It was a fabulous time and even though I had only been away four days it felt like two weeks, we packed so much into our time.

I would like to do a sponsored walk for Cancer Research in September – it's called Shine Walk, as it takes place during the night around the illuminated landmarks of London. I will post on FB the details should anyone want to sponsor me – or come and join. The more the merrier. I will walk in memory of all those amazing people I have known killed by cancer and of course in the hope that money raised will stem the tide.

My hand is forced... honest

2 JANUARY 2015

Blame Fen. She thinks I should continue to blog. I can send out her contact details should you wish to pen a complaint. Her reasoning is that a) it gives me something to do (fair deal), b) I enjoy it (quite), and c) other people enjoy it (hmmm).

So here it is. I am contemplating writing another blog entitled 'ennui'. I confess that I am in limbo. Not dissimilar to Dante's limbo where souls are tormented with endless time doing nothing and no way out of it. That's me at the moment. This isn't some pity piece, I promise, but right now just a statement of fact. If I do write the other blog, I think I want it to inspire – me and others. I am contemplating setting myself a challenge to learn something new every day or to do something different every day. I don't mean take up particle physics or Mandarin but actually using my brain and engaging myself in breaking my routine.

I would love some suggestions and challenges – but they have to be free, i.e. cost nothing, as one of the main reasons that I am stuck is that I am broke. Literally and figuratively. So if it involves buying something or travelling somewhere that's off the radar until I start earning some money.

I have thought about selling a kidney but quite frankly mine are both pickled and also probably damaged by chemo so that's not going to work. I could sell my body but at my age I a) can't be bothered with the upkeep necessary to allow oneself to show any flesh – that personal topiary routine of the pubes, let alone the deforestation of the limbs and then there's the lighting to consider – how to attractively light dimply flesh in an era of too-bright LCD and eco bulbs (where the minimum is way over that old fave of 40 watts dim) and then b) there's the complete lack of any kind of sex drive. I am a little disconcerted by the latter as in my day I really enjoyed sex but now I can think of a hundred things I would rather be doing than any kind of sexual gymnastics. It's not because my body is now scarred after various operations but that my body is just not willing to be involved in that way any more. I am not even sure if the one time I had sex this millennium was actually memorable or enjoyable or just momentous. Could it be the lack of practice or just the lack of patience? Either way, selling my body would not be lucrative – it would have to be discounted and that would be just too depressing for words.

Another friend suggested eBay, not for sex, mind you, or for selling my body, but for everything else. She sells her clothes – but on looking through my wardrobe I am just not sure who would want amorphous, mainly black, baggy cardigans and shapeless trousers? Perhaps there is a market for clothes to make you look invisible. I do worry that I have become that invisible middle-aged woman hiding in her shapeless M&S easy-care range. I do have great underwear but I won't be selling that on eBay. I have probably said it before, but underwear is very important. Even if you hide it under the aforementioned shapeless easy-iron pull-on leisure wear, you cannot go out without good underwear – what happens if you are run over? At least the paramedics picking up my entrails from the tarmac won't be appalled that I didn't make any effort in the bra and knicker department. (I am certain that that will be the first thing on their minds.)

So if it's not selling my kidneys or my body, that leaves my brain and my experience – both of which seem to be a major obstacle to me getting any kind of work. I was encouraged from a very young age to use my brain. My father lied and told me that a good education and plenty of hard work was what everyone would want in the future. Bollocks. Sorry. But it is awful to think that only two generations on from the suffragettes and the pioneering women of the post-war era that we women are not all sitting at the top of the food chain – running FTSE 100 companies and countries. I feel like I want a refund.

My very first job (apart from the part-time tour guiding) was just after I had graduated from university with a very good degree and arrived in London à la Dick Whittington bar the cat. It was the late eighties and the shoulder pads and double-breasted suits spilled out of every champagne bar and posh 'bistro' in the city. Eager beaver that I was, I immediately went to the nearest temp agency – which was called Office Angels and was on Tottenham Court Road. They asked me my qualifications: thirteen O levels, two A/O levels, four A levels, two S levels and a First Class Honours degree. They looked aghast. It seemed I had no USEFUL qualifications. They showed me several photos of telephone switchboards and asked me if I could use any of them. No. Could I use a computer? A what? Could I file? Of course. But I failed their filing test and I was deemed 'unemployable' by Office Angels. As it happened, though, a few days later they called to say they had a job that fitted my poor skills base. I reported to Amoco, the oil company, and was given a hundred coloured pencils, a map of what it looked like five miles under the seabed and a colour code, and I was to colour it in. A skill I learned at kindergarten. Perhaps I should have stayed in that job after all – I would have a wonderful knowledge of colour charts.

This last year, apart from finishing radiotherapy (hurrah), making some films for Breast Cancer Awareness and running a three-day workshop for Aussie producers, I don't know where the time has gone or what I have done with it. I seem to have developed a new skill – filling in time. As Northcote Parkinson said – an alumnus of one of the schools I went to – work fits into the time allotted to it. So WTF have I been doing with my time? Obviously not personal grooming... I just can't think.

To stop this pattern continuing I need a project. I will start tomorrow (the traditional day for all diets and projects) and think about a new skill or challenge for each day as well as more ingenious ways to pay the bills.

Happy New Year

x

H is for Hawk, B is for...

29 JANUARY 2015

H is for Hawk is the winner of the Samuel Johnson non-fiction prize and is apparently a story about a woman coming to terms with a tragic event in her life by working with a hawk. Not sure this method will help me and anyway I am not so sure about raptors. After all, according to *Jurassic Park* they are the descendants of dinosaurs.

But B is for Beaver has grabbed my attention. Yesterday, Natural England gave permission for an immigrant family of Eurasian beavers to stay in their adopted home on the River Otter in Devon. I am assuming that the beavers are refugees from some Eurasian beaver cull and were attracted by the name of the river (perhaps hoping to get it changed to River Beaver) and the charmingly named town of 'Ottery St Mary'. Perhaps these refugees came across from

Calais with the other desperate refugees clinging to Eurostar trains and lorries. What's different, of course, is that the beavers have been welcomed and are now protected. They will have an impact on their environment like any immigrant, and local anglers are worried about the fish in the river if the beavers start damming, but the local town is looking forward to an influx of beaver enthusiasts (oo-er, missus!). It all feels very like a metaphor for what's going on here in terms of the immigration debate. Perhaps if humans grew cute fur and became tourist attractions many in this country would feel more warmly towards them.

My mother's family were immigrants and I don't think we have been too much of a burden on society. Like the beavers they came here to find a better life – escaping Hilter's '*Lebensraum*' greed. But shortly after they arrived they were classed as 'unfriendly aliens' as they heralded from Hungary originally, which in 1939 was part of the Axis powers. Luckily, they were not interned like so many Hungarians, Romanians and German refugees who came to England at that time. But when war broke out they couldn't have radios or cameras. Ironically, my grandfather had been invited here as a civil engineer to work on a social housing project in Leeds (only demolished last year). He spoke German, French, Hungarian and English, and was a devotee of Esperanto, the language invented to be universally spoken so that there could be no more communication problems in the world. There are still people and scholars today who speak Esperanto – which seems to me to be a mixture of Spanish, Latin and German.

My grandfather wanted to help the Allies and every single week for the entire duration of the war he wrote to the Home Office offering his skills as an engineer and his language skills. Typically, he was never taken up on his offer and I still have some of those letters.

They didn't become 'naturalized' Brits until the fifties and when I was thinking about becoming a spy during the dying days of the Cold War my mother's status as 'naturalized' was an issue. Even some forty years after the end of World War Two suspicion about people from 'behind the Iron Curtain' was still prevalent.

My mother had two wonderful friends who had been children like her at the beginning of the war and who had been brought to England on the '*Kindertransport*' trains. They started new lives, integrated and had families, and their stories and experiences, like those of so many other refugees and immigrants, have contributed ineffably to the culture of this country.

I mention all of this as it has been a week of memorials – Holocaust Memorial Day and also the seventieth anniversary of the liberation of Auschwitz. I was amazed to hear and read that the survivors were so ashamed of what had happened to them that many never told their stories for decades. I was also surprised to hear that the actual liberation day was not documented and in fact wasn't acknowledged for days. The Soviet troops, exhausted by their time on the gruelling Eastern Front (and conscripted by Stalin) did not seem especially surprised to find a death camp with its emaciated prisoners. Clearly, life under Stalin had inured them. But also the Germans had fled with the more able prisoners on the infamous Death March across Europe. The initial liberation seems to have been fairly low key and it wasn't until the Americans arrived and started documenting what and who was left that the camp's liberation became news. The Americans later liberated Buchenwald and documented the first person to walk through the open doors.

I was fortunate enough to meet an extraordinary woman called Helen Bamber who only died last year. She spent three years of her life working to repatriate prisoners from Buchenwald. She told me that she couldn't bear the smell of dead geranium leaves as it reminded her of the smell of Buchenwald. I found that one of the most evocative images as hardly a day passes when I don't see geraniums and think of it and her. She was in her early twenties when she started her humanitarian work in Buchenwald and returned to Britain to help set up Amnesty International and continued until the day she died. She established a charity called the Helen Bamber Foundation which works tirelessly to help refugees. Just take a look at the website: www.helenbamber.org.

But what also struck me in listening to the Auschwitz survivors, whose numbers are dwindling fast as most are in their eighties and nineties, was them talking about the importance of culture. One poet would frequently forgo his meagre meal to watch a sunset that would transport him out of the horror of the camp. Musicians would compose and play so that their souls and cultural identity could not be taken from them. But above all a survivor who spoke at the celebration this week said something very important: 'Do not let our pasts become your children's futures.'

For me that says it all . . . oh, and the fact that the beavers have made Devon their home.

Metamorphosis – paws for thought

20 FEBRUARY 2015

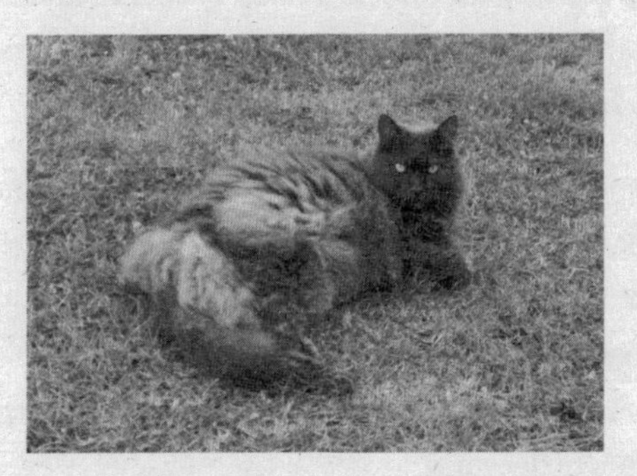

In Kafka's *Metamorphosis* the hero wakes up one morning to find that he has been changed into a large ugly stick insect. I too have realized that gradually I have turned into my cat. I am not yet eating my meals on the floor (standing up at the kitchen counter) and I haven't yet found a way of licking myself clean but I have started to inhabit his world completely. Whenever I am lost for something to do I go to bed (he manages around eighteen to twenty hours a day, I survive on a little less). If I am feeling really adventurous I go into other rooms and then the garden, just like him. Who is emulating whom?

Grably is sixteen-plus years old – in human terms that makes him around eighty-two. He was never particularly adventurous or energetic and so the deterioration in his routine has been almost imperceptible. He has the run of all of the rooms in the flat. Sometimes he sleeps in my bedroom (alternating between pillows, floor, chairs, etc.), sometimes he sleeps in the spare room, sometimes in the study. He hangs around the open-plan kitchen-dining-lounge area when he is hungry (most of the time) or feels he needs to pay me some attention – mostly so that he can get fed.

He has shown no interest in the bathrooms – at one time I did consider teaching him that pointless and obnoxious trick of cats using human toilets but a) who can be bothered and b) if I had he would probably want to use it at the same time as me and, as in everything, he would take precedence.

He does go out into my lovely back garden but does not stray into neighbouring gardens or climb trees, chase birds or annoy squirrels – he is very zen. In my old cottage in Kensington (doesn't that sound poetic?) he wandered around through the neighbourhood and I suspect got fed by other mad cat ladies, but here he is content to inhabit this little world.

My cottage (all sounding very Hollywood right now) was not nearly as ideal as it sounds. It was a two-up two-down (rooms, that is) built in the 1870s on an estate commonly called the 'button' estate. This wasn't some kind benefactor who had made his money in buttons but rather a social housing project for workers who wore buttons on their uniforms – policemen, fire wardens, nurses, etc. The estate was charming; each street was slightly different in design and included corner houses with turrets. The streets were laid out in a grid pattern – north to south were numbered Sixth Avenue, Fifth Avenue (not quite as chichi as the eponymous Manhattan address) and so on, but curiously there was no First Avenue and the cross streets were named by the local bigwigs, some using their own names and others marking a historical event. One street was called Oliphant Street – I understand that this wasn't a misspelling of a pachyderm but rather someone's name. I hope to God his kids weren't fat at school.

This would have been the ideal place to spend one's life bar two small niggly factors – location and location. We were the wrong side of Notting Hill and I was on the wrong side of the estate. Just two doors down was the poetically named Mozart Estate. A 1960s social housing project where clearly the architects felt that dingy alleyways and overhead concrete walkways would recreate some Dickensian dream – or perhaps it was a vision of a spacecraft? Who the hell knows? As you can imagine, the dingy alleys and overhead concrete walkways became great spots for graffiti, drug dealing, mugging and even latterly housing Al-Qaeda bankers (I will come back to this). Westminster council cleverly devised a scheme to put all their problem families in an estate as far away from their City Hall as possible and shoved them into the Mozart Estate. The police would only visit in heavily armed packs – even after a bit of a refurbishment which saw the concrete walkways knocked down and new lighting put in.

So the 'button' estate (cute Victorian cottages) and the Mozart Estate – (gun-toting, high-on-drugs criminals) lived side by side and in my case quite literally so. The house next door to mine was fire-bombed by a rival drug gang... luckily I wasn't at home but some very nice fireman with awfully big feet broke in to save my pad. Even ten years later there was still a touch of woodsmoke smell in the upstairs.

My estate had been plundered by the evil Grande Dame of Westminster – not Maggie but her evil doppelgänger Dame Shirley Porter, who decided that she needed to have more votes (Tory) and a cheap way of gentrifying, so her council started selling off the social public houses in nicer areas to get middle-class Tory voters in. This became known as the 'homes for votes scandal' (I'm sure if they had thought harder they could have found a better name). It brought her down eventually and some time down the line I too found myself in one of these houses. I think about 5 per cent of the estate had been sold off by the time I got there.

But I digress – back to Grablypuss. The houses were in long terraces of around thirty properties with interconnecting garden walls. This was a paradise for all manner of pursuits for a large gang of semi-feral cats and some very beautiful Maine Coon males – these are the huge long-haired cats who grow to be the size of a footstool. One evening one of the feral females came in and miaowed so loudly and insistently it was obvious, even to me with no training in obs and gynae, that we were going to have a birth. I had friends round and did the only thing I could think of – dispatched my brother to the local shop for a box, a friend to find old towels and another to boil water (not sure we needed the last – but it's always what they do in films). I sat on the floor and a few somersaults later (cat not me) the first kitten was born. It was an unprepossessing first glimpse of my now life partner. Quite frankly he looked like a sausage that had grown mould – grey and shapeless. Kittens are born blind and their ears are pinned back, so he really didn't look cute, more like something its mother might have sicked up after eating the contents of a hoover.

At forty-five-minute intervals two other kittens were born – black and more kitten-like. And that's how Grably came into my life. Growing up we had had a cat, Mitzi, which was surprising given my father's pathological hatred and fear of them, only slightly tempered by his pathological hatred of the mice we had running round our attic. So a kitten was introduced into a house with a hyperactive toddler and his more lethargic sister, who just wanted to play with it ALL the time. No wonder Mitzi was cantankerous. She showed us all, though, when we all left home. On pretty much the day my brother left, following in my footsteps, my father also packed a bag and left. So naturally the cat felt the burden of filling the human shoes and would sit at the table, on a chair beside my mother, feeding herself using her paws as my mother ate her meal. They even seemed to chat and I swear the cat would even occasionally drop in a human word or two – just to keep my mother wound up on her diatribes against my father (and me). She lasted to be almost twenty and spent many more years at home than I ever did – so all power to her.

Anyway, having only had a female cat I naturally assumed mine were all girls. The grey one (a British Blue/Maine Coon mix) I called Betty Grable because it had such a sassy way of walking. The first visit to the vet revealed two boys and a little girl. And after three long years pretty much confined to this flat, I have definitely started to turn into him. Miaow.

Oh – the Al-Qaeda connection… a few days after the dreadful 9/11 attacks, an area at the corner of my street – literally forty feet away – was cordoned off. Next thing I knew about it was when my mother called to say my house was on the news. It seems that one of the financial masterminds behind the attack lived there for years. I was heartened to think my mother was worried for my safety – not a bit of it… 'That'll bring down the property prices,' she said, helpfully.

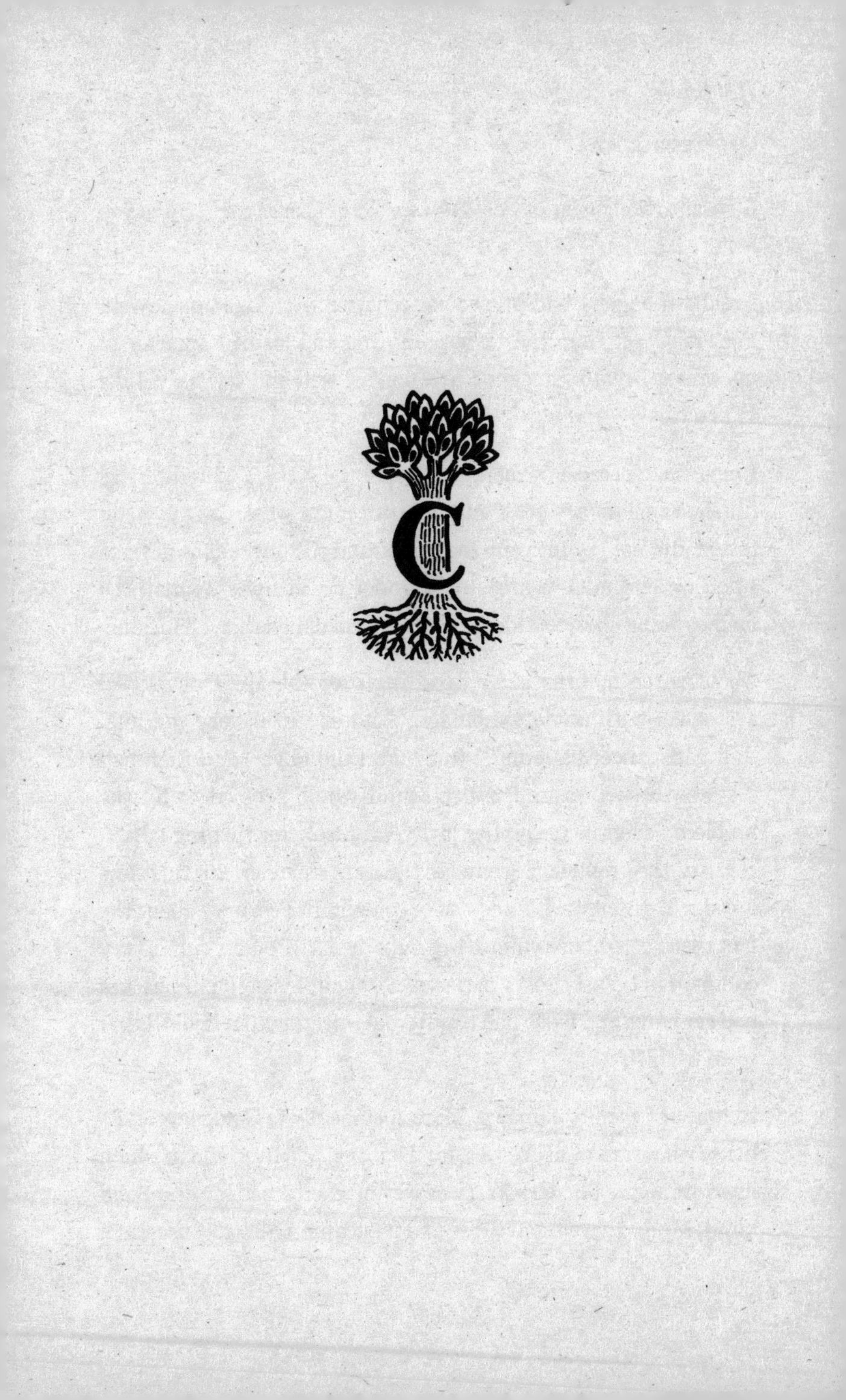

It's back!

6 SEPTEMBER 2015

Like Jack Nicholson in *The Shining*, the cancer is back...can you believe it?

I really thought I had passed cancer with flying colours... well, almost. Apart from the toxic poisoning and losing a quarter of my breast I really thought I had done it well and stylishly. Like I knew...

I have been critical of the aftercare in the NHS. I quite literally finished in January 2014 and up until a few weeks ago I wasn't tested, did not get into any machines and the only examinations I had were of my left breast and under my armpits with all the medics being über-confident that they had nailed this... Hmmm.

About three months after finishing radiotherapy I developed a problem with my left shoulder. 'Rotator cuff is very common in breast cancer patients,' I was told. I did physio and then had a steroid injection under ultrasound which seemed to fix the problem. Then in December last year, just after turning a half-century, the problem migrated to the right shoulder. But this time it did feel different. I asked the oncologist in February about the fact that I could barely move my right arm... 'Rotator cuff is very common in breast cancer patients.' So again I visited physios and had acupuncture. I also had two steroid injections but it just didn't seem to shift.

In March I went to Jamaica. More specifically to Goldeneye – the house where one of my heroes, Ian Fleming, had lived and in which he wrote all the Bond books. I was eleven when I read my first Bond novel. My dad gave them to me and it became a lifelong obsession.

As I mentioned in a previous blog I had always thought I would make a good spy. Admittedly, I saw myself more as Jane Bond than Smiley so when the time came and I got the nod from my Russian tutor I was ready to hide the Walther PPK in my bra and lie back and think of England whilst seducing Russian spies. But the reality as laid out to me was very different. The Cold War was just ending and the role of the spy seemed confined to paperwork. Boring... Where was Goldfinger? Or Pussy Galore?

Since being introduced to Bond I graduated onto Le Carré and also Deighton and any spy books I could get my sticky little fingers onto. But in all the years it was Bond that had taken my fancy. So when my friend Michael decided to spend his sixtieth in Jamaica at Goldeneye I was, as the Americans say, 'made up'. We had a wonderful week sunning ourselves on his private beach where Ursula Andress made her debut in that white bikini, and drinking martinis (well, Jamaican punch and red wine), shaken not stirred on Fleming's terrace.

It wasn't my first trip to Jamaica. I went there first in 2002 at the behest of an international conference on Women in Film and TV. I was already working for a government quango (not a spy although a bloody good cover), and my role was to promulgate international film treaties. I love that word promulgate, it sounds so nasty and dirty. In fact, it just means I laid the groundwork for government lawyers, etc., to draft treaties. It was in that capacity that I found myself in Jamaica, first in Kingston (which I didn't love) and then in Montego Bay (what's not to love). The conference was being run by two Jamaicans who have since become great friends. The first day I arrived to register there was a huge table filled with Jamaican products... No, not that kind. I was particularly taken by the abundance of jerk sauce and happened to comment (aloud) that I knew a few men for whom that would be an appropriate gift and so started my friendship with Fen.

Kate Adie and I were the keynotes at the conference. I love public speaking and by then I was getting into my stride vis-à-vis international speaking jobs. I always liked to start with a joke. In this case I only knew two Jamaican jokes: 'My mother-in-law has gone to the Caribbean.' 'Jamaica?' 'No, she went of her own accord.' Boom, boom. And a more risqué joke: Two men are standing at a urinal – one tall, black and handsome and the other one white, less buffed. The black man looks over and sees the white man has 'Rosie' tattooed on his penis. 'Your girlfriend?' he asks. 'Yes.' The white man looks at the black man who has 'Wendy' tattooed on his. 'Your girlfriend?' he asks. 'No,' says the black man. 'I work for the tourist board. It says, "Welcome to the West Indies and have a nice day."'

Rather oddly I chose to open with the latter joke, which luckily went down well. For even though the conference was 'Women in Film and TV' the audience was mostly men. Anyway, to cut a long story short (sadly there's not time for me to go into my Jamaican adventures, including drinking moonshine with Ms Adie) I had been back to Jamaica many times. Each time I went I got mauled by mosquitoes. My friends there actually started to use me instead of mosquito spray; if we all sat together they weren't bitten as the mossies were feasting on me. One evening I sat outside for about ten minutes and came back with twenty-seven bites. I put it down to me being sweet and delicious, obviously.

So it was of little surprise that I came back from Goldeneye having been bitten by a mosquito or two. Stick with me . . . there is a point to this, I promise.

My friend Vincenzo then asked me to accompany him to Mauritius for a mad six-day holiday. He is trying to visit all the countries in the UN. I have declined offers of trips to Uzbekistan and Azerbaijan but did say I would sacrifice myself to go to Mauritius. Again I came back with several raised welts c/o the Mauritian mossies. Whilst I was there my right arm became increasingly useless.

Just before heading off there I had seen the oncologist. I had had problems getting onto the bed to be examined as I was having very strange aches and pains in my ribs and of course the right arm. 'Rotator cuff syndrome is very common in breast cancer patients.' Hmmm.

I had also been to the opticians to get a new prescription for my glasses. I had quite happily lived with my old glasses until my niece pointed out that the text on my phone was 32 points and I still need my specs to read an SMS. The optician did all the things they do: shone lights and made me read the letters on the board at the other side of the room. In the middle of the examination she made a noise that fills anyone with dread. 'Oh...dear...' she said. 'You have dromedaries in your eye.' At least, that's what I thought she said. It turns out they are called drusen, which are deposits on your retina. Yikes. She referred me to the eye hospital for a consultation but not before talking to me about macular degeneration. 'Do I have that?' I asked in fear and trepidation. 'No,' she said very casually. 'I just thought you should know about it.' 'That's like telling someone about HIV when you are looking at their blood test and then saying, "But you don't have it,"' I said. She seemed a bit put out. Clearly she saw her role as a public health info service but it did freak me out.

May arrived. I had sore ribs and a right arm that really didn't work, I was bitten by mossies in Jamaica and Mauritius and I had camels in my eye. The pain was moving to all my limbs. So on the first May bank holiday I called out the paramedics when I couldn't cough, sneeze or sleep without feeling like I was breaking my ribcage. At 4 a.m. on a Sunday morning the paramedics arrived. They checked my vitals and offered up going into A & E but being a bank holiday and all, I would have a long wait with all the drunks, etc. I declined.

On the first working day after the bank holiday I went to see my GP who sent me off for a chest X-ray and blood work. Ten days later they both came back negative. Talking to Fen about it she said it might be chikungunya virus. I didn't make that up, I promise. It is rife in Mauritius and the Caribbean. Carried by mossies, it is a form of dengue which gives you eye lesions (tick), arthritic pain (tick) and general malaise (tick). So that was it. I had a strange tropical virus I couldn't pronounce, henceforth called chicken korma virus. Hurrah, a diagnosis.

I went to Cannes for forty-eight hours during which time I stopped being able to move my lower right arm. Embarrassingly, I had to lift my elbow to shake someone's hand. The pain in my limbs was pretty awful and in general I felt as though I was falling apart.

It got much worse, so bad in fact that the following weekend (another bloody bank holiday, can you credit it) I had to get Greg to take me to A & E at 6.30 a.m. on a Sunday. We were seen pretty quickly by a young junior doctor who started every sentence with, 'Now, what was I going to say . . . ?' which filled us with slight dread. He liked the chicken korma diagnosis although he had never heard of it, despite having just done a tropical diseases rotation. He took blood to be sent off to the Hospital for Tropical Diseases and also looked at the eye lesions. A nurse appeared and said, 'Open wide,' and squirted clear liquid into my mouth. She never said what it was and we didn't ask till much later. It was, in fact, oral morphine. Whilst we waited for the phlebotomy clinic to open to look at the rest of my blood work, the doctor suggested we go for a coffee.

Of course, being very early on a Sunday and also a bank holiday, nothing was open. So Greg gamely trekked off to find a coffee establishment, leaving me on the terrace at the Royal Free Hospital.

The hospital is an ugly concrete affair, built on a hill. The ambulances come in the lower-ground floor, accessed by a road which goes underneath the terrace two floors above. Standing there minding my own business, and if I am honest, tripping off my tits on morphine, I barely noticed a weaselly-looking man reading the *Sun on Sunday*. He came up to me and in a lilting Irish accent asked me, 'So have you decided how you are going to do it?' 'Do what?' I replied. 'Kill yourself, are you going to jump over here onto the ambulances or throw yourself under a bus?' 'Ah, no,' I said. 'That would be messy and anyway I am waiting for a coffee.' He seemed satisfied with that non sequitur and went away. A few moments later he had grabbed my arm and was standing on the outside of the terrace above the road below. I hadn't quite twigged what was going on (morphine brain). A nurse was trying to pull him back and then a chap standing behind me threw me out of the way and wrestled the Irishman to the safe side of the parapet.

By the time Greg got back our wannabe suicider (and murderer if he'd taken me with him) was being pinned to the ground by security staff. 'Did I miss anything?' asked Greg. 'No, not really,' I replied vaguely.

The outcome of our trip to A & E was that the doctor felt I had chicken korma and sent me away with anti-inflammatories. Two days later I went to the GP again. She referred me for an ultrasound.

By mid-June I had seen several doctors and physios and everyone agreed that I had 'rotator cuff syndrome common in breast cancer patients' and possibly chicken korma virus. However, when I did get the ultrasound round about the end of the second week in June, they noticed an anomaly on my ribs. I had three fractures on my right side. Well, that explained the pain but didn't explain why I couldn't account for the damage. No, no one had hit me. No, I hadn't been in an accident. No, I hadn't fallen over drunk, etc.

My GP then smelled that something was not right in the state of Denmark and called my oncologist. So I found myself back in the Macmillan Cancer Centre with my lovely surgeon Jo who had given me the original diagnosis over two years ago. She spent the best part of an afternoon tracking down my blood work at the tropical disease lab which showed no sign of the chicken korma and then very reassuringly and cheerfully said, 'Let's do a CT scan just to be sure.' That was Thursday.

On Sunday I had the CT scan and on Monday morning went to see a chap called the 'shoulder doctor'. We were all supposed to be going on holiday that Thursday, taking a boat round the Greek islands. I was worried that my right arm would be an issue. I was recommended to this shoulder doctor. He charged me a fortune, barely took a medical history. Didn't exam me properly and then said, 'Rotator cuff syndrome, very common in breast cancer patients.'... I know. He then said he could cure me and I would be right as rain for the holiday. Hurrah. It would only cost me another £599 and he could give me a steroid injection right then. OK, I said. (That's what credit cards are for, right?)

That was Monday at 2 p.m. On Tuesday at 10.30 a.m. I saw Jo again at the Macmillan Cancer Centre. I was alone. Absolutely sure that the CT wouldn't have shown anything. I should have twigged that something was up as there were at least three other specialists and nurses in the room. 'There's no easy way to tell you this, Clare. You have incurable bone cancer and the reason you can't move your right arm is that the humerus is fractured.'

Bugger. Bugger. Bugger. Rather stupidly (remember from the first diagnosis I am a cancer moron): 'Can I still go on holiday on Thursday... on a boat?' 'Not a good idea as the tumours (yes, many of them) cause your bones to fracture and a boat isn't very stable, is it?'... Ah, no.

I told her and the others about the 'shoulder doctor'. They saw red and to cut a long story short I got a full refund. I think he received some pretty stern phone calls from the cancer team...

So once again I had to call Greg and tell him to drop everything as I had cancer.

I will continue the story in the next few days. So two years and a month later I had a new diagnosis – incurable bone cancer. Well, that put a spanner in the works.

Dem bones, dem bones

12 SEPTEMBER 2015

'Rotator cuff syndrome is very common in breast cancer patients,' was all I had heard for months. But how about this – which is on every website about breast cancer metastasis – 'In over 70 per cent of breast cancer patients whose cancer returns it is in the bones.'... WHAT...? Yet none of the doctors, specialists, etc. that I had seen seemed to know this.

Anyway, back to day of diagnosis – Tuesday 23 June. 'Clare, you have incurable bone cancer.'... WTF, I think is what the modern kids say... After trying to digest this information I am given a list of immediate tasks:

1. Go to fracture clinic and get sling for right broken humerus.
2. Get humerus X-rayed.
3. Go to Western Eye Hospital for exam to ascertain whether the lesions in your left eye are cancerous.
4. Meet with oncologist team and radiotherapy team in forty-eight hours to discuss next steps – which will include surgery on right arm, and possible shoulder replacement on that side if you don't have enough viable bone. Meet orthopods (not some strange whaling community, as it turns out, but the orthopaedic team) for examination.
5. Don't go on holiday of a lifetime to Greece on a private yacht with family visiting Greek isles.

Armed with the list, I called Greg. Poor Greg – for the second time in his life he had to get a phone call from me saying, 'Drop everything, it's cancer.'... Bloody hell. Greg was about to cycle off to see the dentist to get his left index finger X-rayed... yes, to the dentist. We are a weird lot in our family, clearly. He knew his finger was probably broken. He had damaged it in a cricket match six weeks earlier and now it bent round left-hand corners.

We have a wonderful dental clinic. I am treated by a fabulous and flamboyant Tenerifian supermodel called Sandra. Greg is treated by a much less flamboyant chap. He wants to change to Sandra, of course. Our previous dentist was Tom the Tooth (our name for him and not his official title). I fell in love with him the minute I saw him. I had just returned from the Australian outback where I had been working on *The Adventures of Priscilla, Queen of the Desert* (now celebrating its twenty-first year). Whilst there we had been in an outback mining town called Broken Hill – because of its slag heap. I developed an abscess on a tooth and the only dentist in town on a weekend was also the vet. He is the only Australian I have ever met who used the word 'strewth', which I had assumed was a Barry Humphries made-up term, but no. 'Strewth,' he said, 'who did this to you?' He was referring to my eclectic collection of implants, fillings, etc. My mother had made me use the dental school, 'because they need the practice,' she reasoned. As our childhood dentist had been called Mr Seaman, it did seem more preferable.

Clearly my dentistry was a mess. On top of that, just before heading out to Australia I had had an unfortunate incident with my jaw. I get TMJ (temple mandibular jaw disease). It means that sometimes it clicks open and other times it clicks shut... so for certain intimate acts (I will spare your blushes) it is like Russian roulette.

When I got back from Oz a friend sent me to see Tom. He looked exactly like David McCallum in *The Man from Uncle* – all floppy white-blonde hair and crinkly blue eyes. He took an X-ray of my mouth and told me I had a hairline fracture in my jaw. 'A sex accident?' he asked. How did he know? He also had a radio on that was playing a local radio station and it had an article on it about an anti-nausea drug that in six out of ten pregnant women caused them to orgasm as they yawned.

'I can prescribe that,' he said. 'How about you take some and we go to the pub to find the most boring bar fly and test the theory... even though you aren't pregnant.' What's not to love about this dentist, I thought, and so Tom became a regular fixture in my life as he tried and often failed to sort out my terrible teeth. The other thing about Tom was his generosity. Every time he treated me and charged me £50 he would feel so guilty that we would go to the pub and he would order several bottles of wine or champagne. Partly so he could laugh at me trying to drink daintily with a frozen mouth. I must have cost him so much more than I paid him. Sadly, Tom had an accident and lost some of the feeling in his hands and gave up dentistry, so we moved practices.

Back to 23 June. Greg met me at the fracture clinic X-ray department and asked if he could just slip his finger into my X-ray to see if it was broken. To this day (12 September) he still hasn't got it fixed but each time he comes with me to the fracture department he asks about it. Doesn't he know it's all about me?

There was no doubt the humerus was broken. It's called a pathological fracture – psychopathical, I think, would be a better description – it means that it was caused by a tumour and will never heal. Bummer.

At the eye hospital we had to go to the emergency room, which was filled to overflowing with people with red and suppurating eyes. Nice. I felt like I was in an extras casting for *Dawn of the Dead*. The room wasn't huge and the hospital is an Edwardian building on the Marylebone Road. The door to the ER swung open every few minutes as someone new came in. The door not only squeaked, it positively sang like an out-of-tune soprano. This was agony for Greg who knew he could fix it with just a touch of WD40.

There were people of every colour and nationality and of course one chavvy bloke in a track/shellsuit top who was talking very loudly on his phone. He had a Bluetooth thingy in his ear and was looking at his smartphone – where his caller was sending photos of herself in revealing outfits. He shared the news with the room that he liked 'a bit of flesh' on his women. He seemed to have no awareness of where he was or how loud he was being. He was still on his phone when he was called in to meet a specialist. God knows what was wrong with his eyes but he was definitely deaf.

I was sent off to have various machines take photos of the inside of my eye and after about an hour was told I had 'age-related deposits'. The indignity of my aged body depositing stuff all over the place. Isn't there a better way of saying this? At least it wasn't cancer. We went home. Exhausted.

The next few days were a manic round of hospital appointments. The first one was to meet with the oncology team. They reiterated that whilst my cancer was incurable it could be managed and that I would have chemo (no, not again, I groaned – see previous postings on my love of chemo) and some radiotherapy and surgery. First things first, an MRI. Bizarrely, the only way they could get me on the list was to admit me to hospital via A & E in the next few days. So a few days later Greg and I gamely trotted up to UCH's A & E department on Monday night. Even though we were expected it still took four hours for me to be admitted and I finally got onto a ward and into a bed at midnight.

The ward was on the fourteenth floor of the UCH tower at the top of Tottenham Court Road – great views. The section of the ward I was put into was for head and neck cancers palliative care . . . not so great. The A & E team also filled me with morphine and gave me steroids. Those of you who don't know me well don't know that I am hyper enough without giving me steroids but on the 'roids I go manic. My poor oncology team visiting the next morning thought I had had some sort of breakdown. Apparently, not only was I fidgeting but I had only put make-up on one eye. In my defence, I did say I had a broken right arm which makes eyeliner somewhat a challenge and number 2, I was surrounded by dying cancer patients which was making me nervous.

I had the MRI – from neck down to pelvis. I won't reiterate my thoughts on MRI machines – only to say they are very noisy and claustrophobic and I hate them, but they are also amazing in showing your body in minute sections through bones or soft tissue. So about two hours later, eight different doctors sat around the bed talking about next steps. The orthopods were sure there was enough bone to put a metal strut in my arm bridging the elbow to the shoulder – currently it was being held together literally by muscle fibre. They wanted to operate by Friday. They also wanted another MRI to check the arm in more detail. There was also discussion about the tumours (yes, bloody plural) in my spine and whether the neurosurgeons would want to operate on my spine... yikes, and then there were general discussions about the other tumours... others???? Two in my right arm (shoulder and back), several in my ribs and at least three if not more in my spine. Bloody hell, I am covered in the bastards – hereby referred to as 'mets', sadly not the baseball team...

At 7 a.m. on Friday 3 July, having been nil by mouth since the previous evening, we duly reported to the surgery admissions. And waited. And waited. Got seen around three hours later and paperwork was done and I was given the gown, etc., but we still waited. And waited. At 11.30 we were told, 'Sorry, it can't happen today. There was an emergency... Come back tomorrow.' Glad I hadn't put on the paper knickers was my first thought, and then... I am hungry.

This is already a long post so I will pick up the surgery and post-op adventures in the next blog…

Twelve inches

20 SEPTEMBER 2015

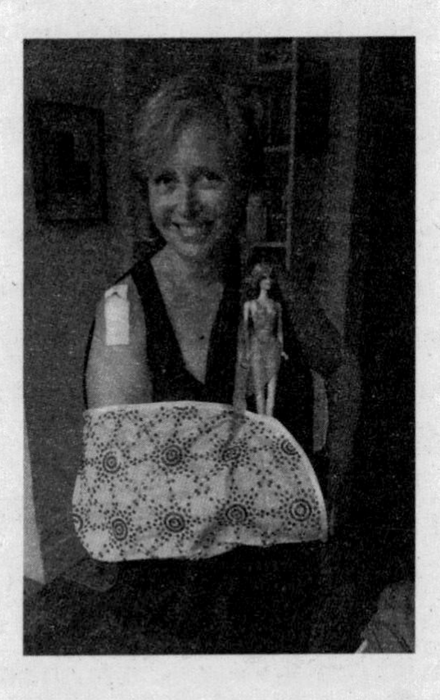

One of the advantages of not having surgery on the 3rd, apart from being able to eat and not being in hospital, was that I could spend time with my friend Sabrina who had just arrived from LA. She had invited me on another yacht to cruise around the Amalfi coast and when she heard that I was in danger of fracturing, she spent a long time fantasizing about getting me a Michelin suit or lots of cushions where I could lie prone on the deck. In the end she decided on getting an avatar – a vintage Barbie with red hair, so she became BC (Barbie Clare) and I could have my holiday vicariously through her. This is a photo of us just after I came out of hospital. BC is the smaller of the two Titian-haired dolls…

Anyway, the following day I did get to put on the paper knickers, gown and long socks and was taken to pre-op. Because I had had my lymph nodes out under my left arm I can't have a needle in that arm. And because they were operating on the right, they couldn't use that either. So the anaesthetic, etc., had to be put in my foot.

When I woke up in the recovery room I was quite literally in screaming pain. I had had twelve inches of metal bolted into my right shoulder and elbow to hold the arm together. At first the nurses tried morphine but that wasn't working and they decided to give me ketamine. Some of you reading this won't know that K is a horse tranquillizer. I started to trip. Badly, frighteningly and when the nurse turned into a crocodile and the room was a kaleidoscope they realized that I was not a happy bunny. They had to flush the K out of me and find a substitute – which meant I spent a fair few hours in recovery.

Last time I had a trip like that was with some 'friends' in Dartmoor who helpfully pushed me out onto the moor after telling me there was a murderer roaming the area. Dartmoor is famed for its remoteness and wild ponies and as the mist came down I could hear heavy breathing and panting all around. Thanks, John, Gav and Justin.

This trip was more colourful and less funny. However, I did get through it and ended up on trauma ward. The anaesthetist put a morphine drip in my right foot and I settled into ward life. However, a fellow patient was anything but a peaceful neighbour. She had dementia and as there were no beds in a care facility she had become a long-term patient on the ward. Poor woman screamed and moaned all night long and for a moment I thought I was back on Dartmoor.

I spent three days in hospital and of course the little section I was in became party central. In the bed opposite me was a fabulous lingerie designer and we were soon having fun. We laughed a lot. The morphine helped. Other patients asked to be moved to our section. Greg also provided entertainment and much-needed snacks and food, and waited on us hand and foot. My only real complaint about my fabulous hospital is the food. I ordered a baked potato for lunch and that's quite literally all I got – a plate with a baked potato on it. No garnish or butter or anything.

The orthopods visited, very smug and happy with their handiwork, and I was sent home with morphine and paracetamol. Despite having twelve inches of metal in my arm I have a few very discreet scars – on the shoulder and elbow. Really marvellous work. It is very weird having a piece of metal hold you together. You feel like the Bionic Woman and I am aware of it a lot of the time.

I recovered quite well although I did discover that I am pretty much allergic to morphine as it almost immediately shuts down my kidneys, so I am now on a synthetic morphine. Which no longer causes kidney problems but does stuff me up...

A week later the fracture clinic trimmed the sutures and gave me new dressings and X-rays. They were (and are) very smug with their handiwork. Greg once again tried to persuade them to X-ray his finger but without any luck (there's a theme building here).

I felt so well that the family took off to Scotland but the following day I developed an intense and disabling pain in my upper back near my neck. I had it X-rayed and a large tumour was very visible. The team decided to zap me with radiation – a huge dose. The sort you normally get over a three-week period, but which I had in one dose. They also decided to zap the tumour that had caused the broken arm. Once again I found myself tattooed and slightly sunburnt without having to go on a cheap package holiday. It did put paid to the pain, though, after a couple of days, and gave me a tan mark on my neck.

Em decided she couldn't stay away with me not being well so gave up her holiday to look after me. She instituted a very strict and healthy eating regime (also very tasty) and I started to heal. But of course the best-laid plans of mice and men... let alone me and the team... never go according to plan.

A few days later I discovered that I really couldn't walk. Unfortunately, I found this out in the middle of the night in bed. I couldn't reach the landline or mobile phone so I couldn't call Em who was just a few doors up the road. After a few hours (where helpfully Grably stomped around on my head to encourage me to get up and then tried to push under my shoulder with his head) I managed to inch towards my iPad. I can't call out on the iPad but tried to FaceTime Greg to get him to call Em. Unfortunately, where he was there is no Wi-Fi signal so I couldn't get through. He tried to call me back but I couldn't reach the phone. I was just on the point of FaceTiming or Skyping Esther in Oz when luckily Em arrived. She had had a sixth sense something was wrong.

It took us three hours to get me out of bed and into a sitting position and another few hours to get me a bed in hospital. At first the consultants thought I had fractured my spine. Then they worried I had injured the spinal cord, so once again I went for another emergency MRI. Luckily, there was neither a fracture nor a spinal cord compression but a few of the tumours in the spine and pelvis were causing problems on other nerves. It was decided that I should have another big dose of radiation at the bottom of my spine. But of course it was a weekend and that would have to wait for the following week. Until then I was forced into bed rest and large doses of painkillers.

Once again our little section of the ward became party central, thanks to lovely staff, Em and my fellow patients. The staff were all very respectful of Em until the moment I was discharged and then they all wanted selfies. As most of the staff there are from the Philippines, I suspect that Em is now more famous than Imelda Marcos.

By mid-July I was home again, almost mobile and the team decided that this was the moment for me to get palliative care and to start using the hospice... deep breath, very deep breath. Yes, a hospice. From now on it will be called Club Med (suggested by my friend Franck).

I am running out of space in this section so I will continue on a new page next week.

Clare x

Bones like lace

12 OCTOBER 2015

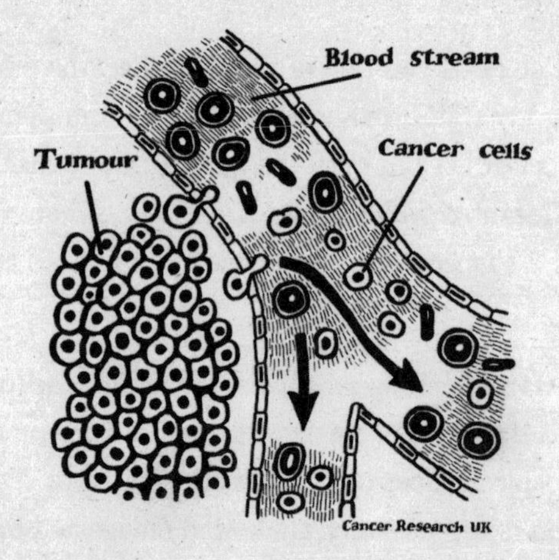

So, what is secondary bone cancer? Well, apparently I still have breast cancer (primary) but I now have bone metastases (secondary cancer)... a lot of bloody tumours in the bones, basically. The cancer moves through blood or lymph nodes into the bones. Bones are constantly growing and shrinking, osteoclasts grow new cells and structures and osteoblasts keep them in check so that they don't grow too much or fracture if the casts don't meet them. As I understand it, the tumours confuse the blasts and casts and they stop doing their jobs, lay down tools and pathological fractures occur. They also make the bones lacey, hence the orthopods wanting to fix more metal to my fraying bones.

That's the science bit. The human bit is that they hurt. A lot. You know that feeling when you get the flu and all your joints ache? It's like that only ten times worse and since there are a lot of bones there is a lot of pain. The painkillers help tremendously, of course, and I couldn't function without them.

When I developed spinal problems the scans showed big tumours resting on nerves and had they been in the spinal cord I would have had to have surgery, but as it was it was decided to blast the bastards with high-dose radiation. Greg wheeled me into the hospital and I was tattooed and sunburnt by the time I got out. On the way back in the cab I got radiation sickness and threw up by London Zoo (with a nice view of the giraffes) and, like a drunk teenager after too many cocktails, I threw up in my handbag as we turned the corner into home. It was like one of those Magaluf hen parties... sunburnt, tattooed, sore and throwing up in my handbag. Add this to the indignity of needing help getting into bed and on and off the loo – well, as you can imagine, I have thrown all self-consciousness out the window.

With Greg away filming, my wonderful, generous friend Jules stepped in to be my carer. I don't think any of my friends ever expected to be helping me on the loo let alone everything else. Jules and Rose were brilliant and, as mums themselves, they have seen it all. The NHS palliative care team stepped up to the plate and within a few days I had an occupational therapist round to help me 'live independently'. The catalogue she showed me of the goodies I was entitled to was very lowering. Cheerful white-haired elderly men and women in pyjamas and nightdresses were getting in and out of bathtubs with doors on the side, sitting on chairs in the shower and posing beside commodes. Everything was ugly, grey or white plastic. I was not very impressed.

A few days later a commode turned up – very depressing but also very helpful. The team also raised my sofa on blocks and I got two sticks. Yikes, is this how it is going to be?

Greg also borrowed my mother-out-law's bed. (I don't think there is a word for your brother's mother-in-law so I have decided she is my 'out-law' as she is wanted... gettit?) She has a hospital bed that at the touch of a button raises the top or bottom, etc. Greg also arrived with enough climbing rope for me to scale Everest and planks of wood. After a few minutes' hammering and drilling, I had the Heath Robinson of beds with pulleys made from rope to help me move in bed. Very ingenious and eclectic and much nicer than the NHS one in the brochure.

So with my personalized bed, commode and sticks I was able to manage on my own. Grably was very put out by my single-bed sleeping arrangements.

The fabulous head of radiotherapy gave me permission to have a week's holiday in Scotland. The occupational therapist sent a pillow that works on compressed air and at the touch of a button sits me up in bed. There have been a few times in the night when I have suddenly found myself sitting bolt upright in bed and a triumphant-looking Grablypuss with his paw on the controls. We took the pillow up with us. At the airport I had a wheelchair and Greg opted to push it himself, even with his broken finger (still not fixed as I write at the end of September).

We spent a week in good Scottish air and had a very funny obstacle course arranged by the family where Phyllida and I had to compete in races, mental tests and washing-up. Phyllida is eighty-three and it seemed that the race would be evenly balanced. Me with chemo brain and her with old-age forgetfulness... me with a broken arm and her with a genuine frozen shoulder... Needless to say, she won, as the last test was an egg-and-spoon race, impossible with a stick and a broken arm. But we both got prizes and the family had a good laugh at us (and with us) at our expense.

Coming back was tough but the inflatable pillow meant I could have my own double bed back (and fluffy sleeping companion). Since the blast of radiation on my spine I have been able to ditch the commode and although I still need a stick I am so much more mobile. The chemo is really OK as they are no longer trying to cure me, so I get to keep my hair and apart from metal mouth and fatigue it's really not too bad.

I am having a CT scan in early October so we can see whether the chemo is working. We saw my bone scan which made me look like a Jackson Pollock painting – there were so many black dots (tumours). No one has counted them but it's definitely way more than double figures and looked like it was in the twenties to me. So here's hoping that the treatment will have killed off some of those when we see the scan. Onwards and upwards…

Brain scan

16 OCTOBER 2015

I hadn't really thought about my skull but as it is mostly bone I guess it is inevitable that there would be tumours there as well. And guess what…there are.

On Monday 5 October, I was called in for a brain MRI. There are some word combinations that excite you – 'upgrade to first class', 'sunny and warm' etc. – and some that are horrid combos – 'spinal surgery', already mentioned to me a few times, and 'brain scan' – yikes.

This all came about when last week I got sick with what felt like the flu. By Friday I was shivering uncontrollably so had to go to the hospital and was put in an isolation room in the haematology department. They took my vitals and then took blood. Forty-five minutes later they came back to take more blood, and again an hour later. It seemed that they kept losing my blood, not very reassuring in a department that specializes in blood.

The doctor wanted to admit me to hospital but we (Greg was there as my brilliant support team, as always) decided to renege on that and went home. At 10.30 that night the registrar rang to say that they had lost the last lot of blood and unless I felt awful I should stay at home, but that I had to come back on Monday for a brain scan. It seems that shaking can be an indication of a brain tumour.

On Monday I went for said MRI. They strapped me into the machine, put a mask over my neck and face, and gave me earphones. I was there for almost an hour. The machine as previously noted is loud and claustrophobic and the music was a selection of German classics – Wagner, mostly. The last five minutes or so was variations on Haydn's theme of '*Deutschland Über Alles*', definitely not what you want when you are already feeling uncomfortable. I suggested to the MRI team that they needed to change their classical music selection as the German national anthem was not exactly relaxing.

I followed my MRI with a CT scan of neck to pelvis. Much easier to cope with, and then I had a two-hour meeting of the Cancer Patients Advisory board on which I sit... UCH is building a new state-of-the-art cancer facility and I am helping them with bits and bobs and trying to raise money for a proton beam therapy machine which I hope will be my legacy. More about the machine in a later blog.

Today, Tuesday, my oncologist has told me that the tumours in my skull are pressing on the brain lining and she will have to consult with the neurological team about next steps. They may suggest radio to zap them but I am a little worried about frying my brain. We are meeting with the team on Thursday to see if the CT scan shows progress on the chemo front and to discuss my brain. I have to be honest, I am pretty freaked out right now.

On another note my faithful old (fifteen-year-old) Apple laptop finally gave up the ghost today. I took it to the Mac shop to get a new battery and realized that not only were most of the sales assistants in nursery school when I bought the machine but also no one replaces batteries any more. So I was forced to get a new machine. The sweet sales guy offered an extended five-year warranty on the machine, but I declined. I didn't feel it should have a better life insurance policy than me.

Sorry, this blog is a bit of a downer but I am sure it's just a temporary blip. I am quite fond of my brain and the thought that it might be fried is a little overwhelming. I promise normal black comedy will be resumed in due course.

x

What the oncologist said

20 OCTOBER 2015

My bones are looking a lot better – although the CT scan is very difficult to interpret as most of my tumours were 'lytic lesions' (holey... not God-fearing, but like Emmental cheese) which means that the bone looks like it has been eaten away. The chemo has made them sclerotic, which means denser. They are easier to see and much less painful.

I have several fractures in my spine but they are not planning to do anything about them unless I am in pain, in which case they will zap them with radiation (a 'welding job', as my friend Ruth calls it).

The skull MRI shows diffuse tumours – no big lumps but the only concern is the one on the right parietal bone and dura (it goes bone/fluid/dura/fluid/brain). That's just above the right ear. My understanding is that damage to that area – should it get worse – will affect my ability to dress or wash and hamper me from constructing things or painting. Phew, none of those seem to be fundamental to my day-to-day living so that's not too bad. Washing is overrated and I am crap at DIY and art therapy has been a disaster.

They are not especially concerned about this, although they have made an appointment for me to see a neurosurgeon in a couple of weeks' time. The tumours are not in the brain tissue and won't jump from bone to tissue there.

I had to ask for a prognosis. Clearly, this is an inexact science and I am only a few months into treatment which I understand may lose its efficacy as the body gets used to the chemo (what a weird thought). Rather cheerfully the oncologist said, 'A couple of years.'. . . Blimey.

That's obviously an average as some people live longer or shorter than that. Greg reminded me that the consultation was overall good news in the circumstances, even if all I heard was that I would be dead in two years. He remembers word for word a bad review he got for a play at the Edinburgh Fringe over twenty-five years ago. He can't remember any of the positive reviews.

I am not going to dwell on the bad, but concentrate on the good. If the current chemo stops working, they have other chemo options and endocrine treatment (whatever that is – I think it may be hormone therapy in which case I may turn into Bruce Jenner). I am fired up to beat the average and be here to irritate family and friends for longer than two years.

Still . . . my heart did stop but I didn't cry . . . I am only human, after all.

x

Accentuate the positive

23 OCTOBER 2015

A million years ago (figure of speech, of course, as this is not an anthropological posting) Rose gave me a mixed tape. It was very much something we all did – if there was a boy you fancied you might do him one, or vice versa, and each song always ended with the familiar clunk of the pause button on an old tape recorder. But they were very special. On one such tape, Rose chose the Bing Crosby version of 'Accentuate the Positive, Eliminate the Negative' with the Andrews Sisters as Bing's backing group. The song has been covered hundreds of times by pop stars – most recently, I gather, by Paul McCartney. Anyway, if you YouTube the Bing version there's a very dodgy clip from the film *Here Come the Waves* where Bing is blacked-up to sing it. That reminds me of when I introduced my Rwandan nephew to the fact that we were brought up watching Saturday-night TV which included *The Black and White Minstrel Show*. We thought it was normal for white men to black up to sing jazz songs. I can't believe that this still happened in the 1970s in

Britain. My nephew was both appalled and amused by the clips on YouTube from that show.

This whole thing I'm writing isn't about nostalgia but instead about positivity. After getting my, quite frankly, bleak prognosis, I had a moment. Luckily it didn't last too long. The following day the sun was shining and I felt very positive. I spit in the face of this prognosis and laugh the average statistics out of the window. I am NOT going to focus on something I can't control and instead focus on something I can . . . my well-being.

I have been a bit Pollyanna-ish before and I apologize to anyone who misses my deeply cynical side (it is still there, I promise) but I am really starting to believe that I can not only help myself but that being positive and being surrounded by love and joy will help. Obviously not twenty-four hours a day as I would quite seriously end up murdering, but you know what I mean.

When I first visited Mumbai I was fortunate to stay at the sumptuous Taj Mahal Hotel by the Gateway of India. On my first morning I was fixated by a group of (mostly) elderly people gathered in a circle in front of the Gateway with their hands on their hips laughing uproariously. They were the Colaba Laughter Group. They meet every morning at just after sunrise and standing together they laugh and laugh and laugh. They absolutely 100 per cent believe that this cures ailments and keeps them young. I must say none of them dropped dead whilst I watched them over a period of a week so there must be something in it.

I read about a woman in the US who when faced with a similar cancer prognosis decided to have at least five minutes twice a day of unbridled fun with her daughter. This grew into her setting up the Comedy Cures Foundation (www.comedycures.org) which seems to organize people to come round and cheer you up, make you laugh and make you feel better. She has outlived her prognosis by at least fifteen years. I have no idea if something similar exists in the UK and I know I would freak out if a clown turned up on my doorstep but hey, whatever works. We have a saying here that 'laughter is the best medicine'... and maybe it is. Ha ha.

I am reading a lot around cancer and complementary healing, which I did not do the first time round. I am not very good at self-help-type books and in the past have used them mostly as a wedge under wobbly furniture. However, at some very fundamental level I am a believer that you are what you eat and if you go through life only seeing the negative that is what you will see. So in my own way I am open to anything holistic and my doctors are very encouraging about it. I do not see the 'alternative' treatments as that, but do see them as complementary. With this in mind I have been exploring the possibility of other holistic approaches and recently met with a doctor from Bangalore who runs a clinic there which looks after the whole body, medically, spiritually and emotionally. I am thinking of going there for a month in February with the blessings of my onco team, etc., I am very excited as I love India and I want to learn meditation and about myself. Karnataka is where Ashtanga yoga came from three thousand years ago and Ayurveda, so I feel I am going to the right place.

On the medical front I have seen the Club Med doctors and also the orthopods about possible surgery. Nothing has been decided about preventative surgery on my femur even though I have a fracture there. I am seeing the neurosurgeon on Tuesday about the skull tumours and my spinal fractures. All I want is to be able to travel to India, do some yoga and yogic breathing, etc. etc.

I have been treated all the way through in Reiki by my lovely friend John (an ex-model). There are photos of him in the first cancer treating me during chemo. He has been amazing (as have all my friends) and he was treating me this morning and my cat was sitting on my head all the way through just monitoring John and where his healing hands were going – clearly ready to pounce and kill. And then this afternoon I was reading in one of the cancer books that pets are as healing as laughter. Now all I have to find is a laughing cat.

'Toodle-oo…'

27 OCTOBER 2015

Went to the Royal Neurological Hospital yesterday to meet with an onco-neurologist, ostensibly to talk about my skull tumours and fractures in my spine. Thank goodness Greg was with me, otherwise I would have thought it was a bad comedy show and would have been looking for the hidden camera.

It was bizarre and very funny…not what we were expecting. The chap we saw was OCD. We were ushered into this very unprepossessing room by the consultant, who was lanky and with shocking teeth. There was a young student in the room on what we thought was work experience. The consultant had lined the chairs up at a 45-degree angle to him, as though we were there for a recital or something. Doctors in my experience tend to want you to sit by their desks and within reach, not halfway across the room in an audience formation. Anyway, this chap asked about my symptoms and as I spoke he kept closing his eyes and looking like he was about to fall asleep. He then wanted to examine my shoulder so I went behind a curtain and, as I was taking off my top, Greg engaged the young student in conversation, who turned out to be around seventeen and still at school and thought it might be interesting to tag along in medicine. Clearly a godson or nephew of Dr Odd.

At the end of the consultation I had learned nothing new about the tumours or location of the fractures and although he had all my scans he looked at them perfunctorily and dismissed them. As we were leaving he shook my hand and then said, 'Toodle-oo.' Twice.

Greg and I were clutching each other trying not to laugh. It was, quite frankly, surreal and bizarre. Who says cancer can't be funny?

A new design and almost a new me

23 NOVEMBER 2015

Sorry it has taken me so long to update but I am a computer idiot and so had to be retrained in how to use my website. As Homer Simpson would say, 'Duhh.'

Everything is almost tickety-boo. If it weren't for the cancer I would be really well. I feel pretty good – have a new trendy pixie haircut (courtesy of my sis-in-law) and have managed to make it through another birthday – fifty-one is such an ugly number, a horrid prime that is neither attractive nor useful. All it means is that I have made it into my fifties so I guess I should be grateful for small mercies.

I am now in a regular cycle of two weeks' oral chemo and a week off and am about to start my eighth round. No idea how long this will all last – I guess until my body gets too used to it all. I am pretty mobile but hate the cold damp English autumn weather. When people say they feel the cold in their bones I now fully understand the saying.

My bones feel cold and that doesn't seem to go away no matter how much I heat my flat. In an ideal world I would be a winter bird – flying off to warmer climes the moment the temperature wavered around single digits and arrive back here in time for the beautiful late spring.

However, until I sprout wings and until my travel insurance allows me to go to more exotic (warm) places, I am a little stuck to Europe. Jules is taking me to Majorca this weekend though and hopefully we will catch some late sun. I can't wait. I have never been and am excited. We won't be going to Magaluf but to more sedate parts. Even though I already have several tattoos I am not ready for Magaluf.

I had a bit of a bad week just before the old birthday. I dream of being independent for as long as I can. This includes financial independence. My gorgeous family have been keeping me afloat – as Greg says, it will all come out in the wash (meaning 'The Will'). But I have a pension plan that it seems likely I may not live to be able to cash in. It seems crazy to me that this is MY hard-earned money but according to the HMRC website I can't get it unless I promise to die within twelve months. Harsh or what?

So I trooped off to see a financial adviser to try to understand if there was any way round this. It was a most depressing ninety minutes, worse than my prognosis. He meant well but spent forty-five minutes telling me in great detail about his wife who had died of the same cancer. (Why do people do that? If I bought a yellow car no one would tell me about their experiences with a yellow car but for some reason if you have cancer some people want to tell you about their horrible and always fatal experiences.) After the uplifting story about her death, he then said the only way I could get my money would be to get my oncologist to write and say I had less than twelve months to live. When I objected (I do not want to see that in writing and anyway, I don't believe it applies to me) he said, 'My wife would have done that.' As you can imagine I was screaming at the top of my lungs (internally) and left there feeling broken and depressed. He offered to write to Greg so that he could make the choice for me. For God's sake, I am a well-educated woman who can make decisions for herself. He also introduced me to a lawyer who would do my will. It just got more and more cheery.

It took me a week to slough off (is that the right spelling – should it be 'sluff'?) the feeling of impending doom. I spoke to the pension people who were lovely but the bloody law says if you cash in your pension before you are fifty-five you either have to die quickly (and not get to spend the money) or pay an arm and a leg in tax and since my arm and both legs are fractured I doubt whether HMRC would want either.

Oh, well. It's only money and I need to concentrate on positive thinking and staying well. So two fingers up to the HMRC and depressing financial advisers – hurrah for gorgeous friends and family. I'm off to Majorca to score me a wealthy ex-pat. (I hope he won't want jiggy-jiggy as my pelvis is too fragile for that…)

xx

To India and beyond

26 JANUARY 2016

The funny thing about being in a wheelchair at an airport is that the minute you sit down you clearly also don your cloak of invisibility.

No one actually talks to you. They talk to the person pushing you (who unless it is a family member is a stranger you have met five minutes before): 'Can she walk up steps?' for example, was what one personal service person asked the man pushing me. 'I am here and reasonably coherent and can answer for myself,' I wanted to shout but of course being the good English patient I didn't scream at the top of my voice or even yell. I merely waited for him to look down and ask me. Have I bought into the helpless cripple routine already?

I used to travel a lot. I mean, a lot. I was in Heathrow at least four or five times a month, sometimes twice in one week. I never ever considered being anything other than a truly independent traveller. I arrived with just enough time to get through fast-track customs, security, grab a bite in the lounge and get on the plane. I don't think I ever for one moment thought about someone less able than me and how they managed. Most airports are huge. The chap pushing me at Stansted from my Ryanair flight to the exit told me it was a mile between the two. Most of that mile is shopping. In all the years I flew I never thought I would be anything other than someone who could always just manage for themselves.

Only once was I brought up sharp and that was when a chap next to me on a plane to Dar es Salaam via Nairobi died. That was a reality check for sure. It was in the days when you could still smoke on planes. He, his wife and I were sitting in a row just in front of the area you could smoke in. He was French. About four hours before landing in Nairobi he had a breathing problem. None of the cabin staff on the BA flight spoke French even though Dar es Salaam was once under European rule. Anyway, we laid him out at the back of the plane and got oxygen. They tannoyed for a doctor but there wasn't one – there was a dental hygienist, not really something he needed at that time. They administered oxygen whilst in my terrible school French I tried to ascertain his symptoms and medical history. Several people got bored of waiting for a fag whilst the oxygen was being used and they started smoking. It's a miracle we didn't explode.

So there he was lying at the back of the plane in a fog of smoke dying beside a broken lavatory. Not pleasant. Sadly, he died and all they did was cover him with a blanket at the very back. There was an ambulance waiting at Nairobi and that was that. When I got back to the UK I wrote to Lord King (former chair of BA) to complain. I got back a voucher for £150 which could only be used against a full-fare flight (needless to say I still have it) and a short note apologizing for the inconvenience caused. Bloody hell.

Hardly a response worthy of 'the world's favourite airline'...

Anyway, just to reassure you all, we got to India without a hitch. And we are now ensconced in this fabulous vortex called the International Centre for Holistic Health.

Tantalizingly, I am not going to write about being here in this post as I have to be up for yoga at 6.30 a.m. and I need my beauty sleep. Tune in later.

x

I have a chaste tree and a drongo in my garden

13 FEBRUARY 2016

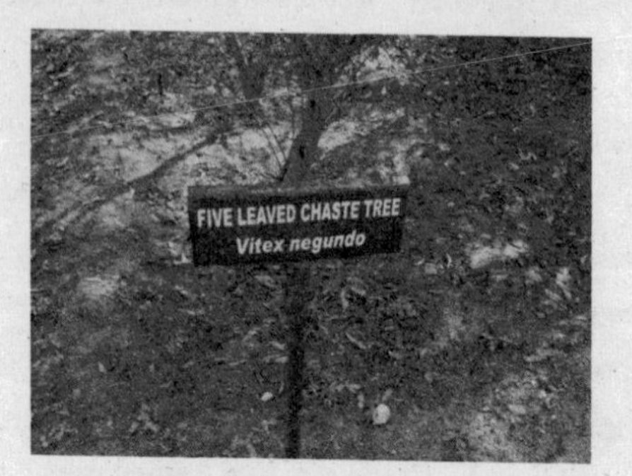

I feel like I have landed in an Edward Lear story. I have never heard of a 'chaste' tree . . . somehow I never expected trees to be rampant sexually or priapic (apart from in appearance). Anyway, this tree is apparently *Vitex agnus-castus* which in its homeopathic form takes away any sexual desire – it's an anaphrodisiac. Laughingly, it is also prescribed to menopausal women . . . like we need anything to persuade us against sex at this time. The drongo is a big black fork-tailed bird with a lovely song. Of course, the word has different pejorative meanings, especially in Australia.

I am sorry I haven't been posting but weirdly I have been busy. I know that sounds odd, especially as I am at a clinic doing mild yoga and having treatments, but it really has been time-consuming.

Arriving here was very funny. We were met off the plane by four young men, each immaculately turned out with pomaded hair and clean pressed shirts and ties, proudly sporting lanyards. It seems nowadays that you aren't anyone unless you have a lanyard. I see people wearing them on the Tube as if to say, 'Yes, I have a job that needs a lanyard.' I would rather die than wear a lanyard outside of conferences/film festivals where it was mandatory. But back to our welcoming party. They were as keen as mustard and reminded me of the students I see on *University Challenge* here in India. It's a hugely popular show and the students wear ties and take it very, very seriously.

Having picked up our bags we emerged into the cold foggy Bangalore early morning when a young lady rushed at us with a bunch of red roses. Poor Em, I thought, even here she can't just blend in, but as it turned out they were for me. So there I am in my wheelchair with four attendants and a posy on my lap having my photo taken. I felt very strange.

Soukya is on the edge of Bangalore, the fastest-growing city in India. It wasn't on the edge of the city when Dr Mathai established it fifteen years ago. Then it was surrounded by fields and farms. Now every day the city is creeping closer. There's a railway line that runs along the compound. When they started building the clinic there was a freight train every other day and the odd passenger train. Now the trains clatter past at all hours of the day (and night), hooting their horns vigorously. At first I thought it might be to put two fingers up to the pampered rich folk in the clinic who are supposedly observing silence in meditative states but actually it is because people walk along the train tracks and also sleep on them. The hooting is to wake them up. It certainly wakes me up. At first it felt like the trains were about to come hurtling through my room and my dreams were of *Eraserhead*, but now I am getting very fond of them.

The actual compound is an oasis of tranquillity and beauty and is full of birds and exquisite flowers. There are also animals and all the vegetables cooked here are grown here. It is really very paradisal (or maybe slightly cultish as the patients walk around in cream silk PJs for yoga?).

On our second day a baby goat was born. I saw it minutes after it was born, still covered in goo. A couple of hours later I took Em to see it and it was still covered in goo and by itself in the pen. All the grown-up goats had been taken out for grazing. In typical Western (urbanized) way both Em and I were appalled and rushed to reception to complain about animal cruelty. To say that the receptionist was gobsmacked by our demands that the farmer returned the mother immediately, would be an understatement. We definitely looked like two hysterical middle-aged Hyacinth Bouquets (reference to a TV show about a middle-aged fusspot). A few hours later the farmer, looking rather nonplussed, showed us the baby goat clean and happy . . . phew.

However, a short while later I was walking past and the baby seemed immobile and I rushed at the farmer again, but it was only asleep. So henceforth the goat born on day two here has been called Lazarus.

Later that same day Em and I were walking the compound when we came across a bird caught in the netting for the grapes. We came back to the room and grabbed nail scissors (and rather inexplicably, also tweezers – what was I going to do, pluck it free?) and also gloves. Em pointed out rather sadly that the gloves were less than useless against the bird's sharp beak and claws. Funnily enough, I had not packed gardening gloves or my hawking leather ones! We managed to cut her free and she limped off. She was a magnificent raptor called a koel. So even though we had been stupid about the goat we could congratulate ourselves on the bird rescue.

Apart from wildlife duties – which include me feeding the squirrels and the birds and also hiding from large snakes – most of the day is taken up with treatments. This is my first experience of Ayurveda. 'Ayur' means life and 'veda' means science and it is quite literally that – 'the science or knowledge of life'. It has been practised in India and especially in the south for four thousand years. Of course, the British Raj banned it along with naturopathy, homeopathy and anything that smelled vaguely unscientific to them. But actually, it is scientific and taken very seriously. The doctors here have formal medical qualifications and are constantly doing research into different aspects of it. So this is not just massage with some weird-smelling oils (although it does rather boil down to that in the end).

The basic idea is that in order to heal we need to detoxify and purify (it's called Panchakarma – 'pancha' means five and 'karma' means therapeutic). The massages, enemas and other purgations including washing out the nose and eyes are part of that process. Because I am rather broken and also taking chemo and morphine the detoxification process has mainly been hands-on massages. I don't have to do daily enemas. Phew.

Once the body is detoxified it is ready to heal emotionally and physically. According to Ayurveda, everyone is made up of energies or doshas. When they are out of alignment we get sick. There are three doshas – Vata, Pitta and Kapha – and they have to be in harmonious balance for us to be fit and well. They correspond to body type as well as mental strengths, etc. I am Vata-Pitta, which is normal for a middle-aged woman. So, all the treatments given and the herbs used correspond to recalibrating the balance of the doshas (which my spellcheck wants to put as dossiers).

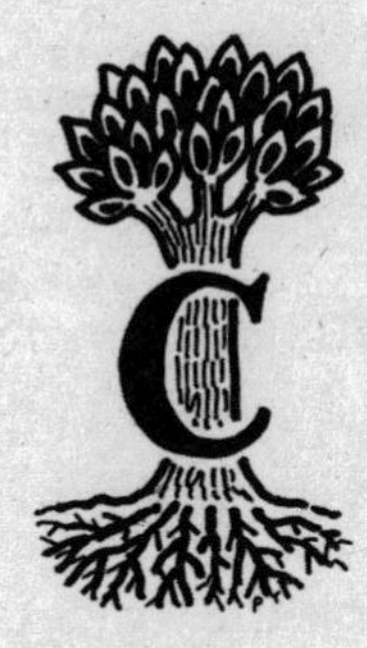

Update

19 JUNE 2016

Apologies, everyone, for the lack of postings. I got back from India in late February to find out that the cancer had spread to my liver and so was taken off the chemo. My oncologist suggested I go on a clinical drug trial which I did for the last three and a half months. Although the idea was exciting in that it combined three different drugs that could cut off the new cancers from growing further, the truth was that the drugs were way too strong for me and I have been pretty poorly. I also hated being a lab rat.

I am now back with the NHS and onto an endocrine treatment and when I have a little bit more energy I will post more. Every day I rally a wee bit but it's very slow progress.

I apologize if I haven't replied to your texts, emails, etc., but I just haven't had any energy.

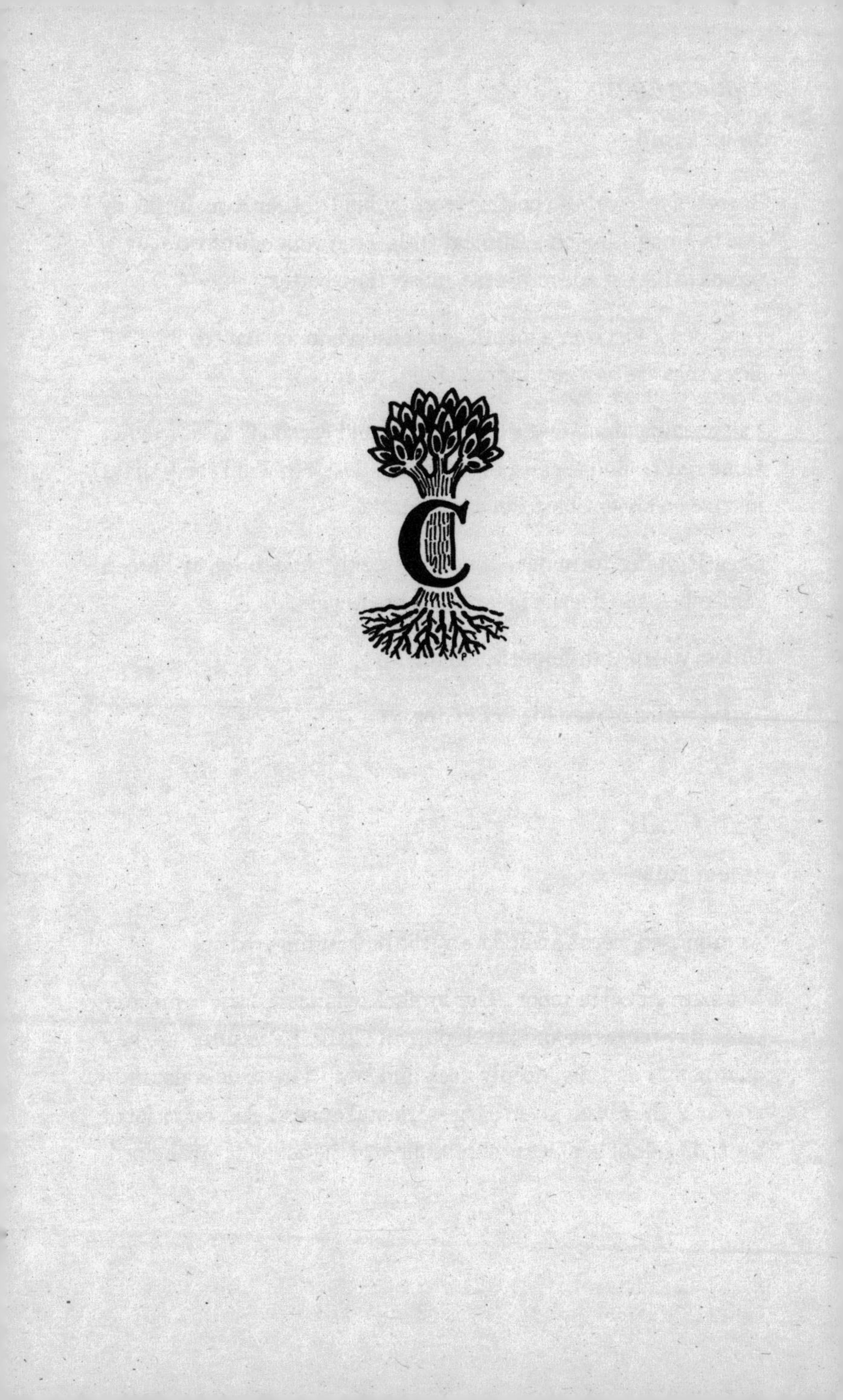

Update again

20 JULY 2016

Sorry not to have been posting recently, but I've been a wee bit poorly due to embarking on a Clinical Drug Trial which, unfortunately, seems to have made me worse, rather than better.

I stopped it just over a month ago and am hoping that the Big Bad-Boy drugs are now coming out of my system.

I also realize that I owe a lot of emails and Facebook messages, let alone return phone calls, SMS, pigeon post, etc. I am sorry that I just haven't been able to do this recently.

Greg is going to update the blog weekly, hopefully, if he can remember, and doesn't break any more fingers.

Unless you hear differently, I'm fine.

Typed with a broken finger by Greg.

Saturday

23 JULY 2016

As promised, here's an update by the broken-fingered one...

Not a great deal to report. Our lovely Kiwi mate, Gary, came over yesterday morning and stuck pins in Clare. He assures me he's qualified to do this. Mainly neck and jaw. Clare feels constantly now as if she's been given a big old dental anaesthetic, and a lot of the right side of her face is numb. She said the acupuncture helped.

Then we went up to the hospice – or 'Club Med'– to have a session with the physiotherapist there. Just finding simple movements that can be done to keep the various muscles functioning. There's not a lot of muscle left on Clare now. We came away with a four-wheeled Zimmer-frame thing: complete with brakes and a seat – we gave it a gentle test-drive in the flat, and I think it'll be useful. Probably most useful on the days we have to leave the flat, especially going into town to the hospital.

Having been out and about yesterday, Clare was exhausted today, so has spent most of the day asleep – unfortunately not listening to the radio, where *Test Match Special* was keeping me afloat – England v. Pakistan at cricket, for those of you not in the know. And a good day for England . . . I kept popping in to see her and feed her watermelon juice, banana smoothies and fizzy water.

She's weak. She sleeps most of the day. Which I can only feel is a good thing – she's at rest; she's not in pain; she doesn't have to keep abreast of Brexit . . .

Thursday

28 JULY 2016

Oops. I got Clare absolutely stoned this morning. My bad. We had been at Club Med yesterday, and the lovely Adrian had prescribed upping some meds that she's on, and introducing others to help with bone pain. He'd typed out a protocol for me to follow, so, in my defence, I was just 'following orders'. . . Suffice to say, we did the morning pill-popping first thing, and by mid-morning she was giving Timothy Leary a run for his money. All good to find out, though – at what point pain control becomes tripping.

So she's had a very relaxed day today.

Not much to report. We are able to dine together every evening – a TV dinner, without the TV, sitting on the sofa munching some nice fresh fish and pasta. I feel like I'm now at least a semi-professional watermelon-juicer – it's a barista for coffee; I wonder if there's a word for a juicer? She now has four litres of it in jugs in the fridge. If you haven't tried it, it's rather lovely.

I'll write when there's more interesting news than drugs and juice…

Gaviscon versus methadone

8 AUGUST 2016

For those of you who don't know, Gaviscon is a liquid relief for indigestion, available over the counter at a pharmacy; methadone is, according to the Internet, 'a powerful synthetic analgesic drug which is similar to morphine in its effects but less sedative and is used as a substitute drug in the treatment of morphine and heroin addiction'. Not a lot of crossover there, then. Apart from on Clare's bedside table: Gaviscon right next to her (as she finds it soothes her tummy), and the methadone on the far side, the bottle in a mug with a 5-ml syringe to administer the correct dose. A couple of mornings ago, I wandered in about 10 a.m. to check on her and discovered, once again, Timothy Leary's little friend – she'd had a bit of a tummy ache, when half asleep, and for some reason had over-reached…

The methadone is now in another room.

Quiet days, still. Some better than others. Some lovely moments, such as yesterday, when Clare managed for the first time in many days to get to the sofa for dinner, whilst I changed her bed-linen for a beautiful, new, soft, Egyptian cotton set that her lovely friend Fiona had just bought. Now, obviously, covered in cat hairs...

We are hoping for a visit this week from the occupational therapy crowd, to see if there are any new gadgets we can have to make life easier. Clare is fantasizing about having a bath, so we can maybe get an electric bath chair thing, that raises up and down and tips, so you can lie back and soak. I'll keep you all posted.

Grably Puss

11 AUGUST 2016

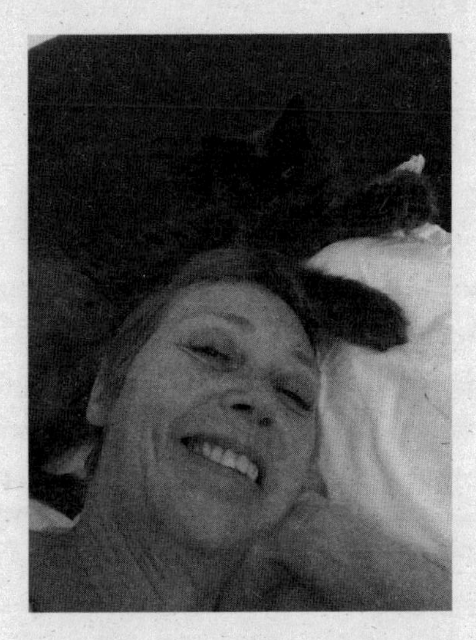

Grably Puss. Probably spelt wrong. The name of Clare's cat. Born, as she likes to tell the story, on her lap, some seventeen years ago this September. A big, fluffy grey thing, even at birth, and assumed to be female. And thus named Betty Grable. After the film star. Goodness only knows why... And then, after some time, it was discovered that Betty Grable had testicles. A quick name change thus ensued to 'Betty Gray-balls', which, over time was reduced to Gray-balls, and then Grably Puss.

Recent cat-sitters for Clare, who came to stay when she would go overseas travelling, misheard the name, and gave him the moniker 'Gravy Puss'.

There is some sort of reason why I am sharing this, as I am in a constant state of bemusement with our furry friend, as I will feed him his sachet of cat food, and within seconds he will be headbutting me for a second helping. A more forensic look at his almost-still-full bowl, shows that he now merely licks the gravy from the meat or fish. Gravy Puss he is, then...

Apologies to the cat

12 AUGUST 2016

On telling Clare this morning about the blog posting I wrote saying the cat was about to be seventeen, and was Clare going to have to pay for his driving lessons, I was reliably informed that he will turn eighteen on 2 September. Thus will want as a present a downpayment on an apartment. Apologies to the cat...

Big day today. We had the occupational therapist, Nicola, here in the morning, helping me to work through what bits of kit would be useful now for Clare. And this is why I keep banging on about why we should all gladly pay our taxes (for those of you who don't know, I made a documentary for British TV at the start of the year about tax avoidance/evasion) – Nicola left us just before noon, and by 8 p.m., we had delivered to our door: a wheelchair thing that has a hole in it, so you can wheel it above the loo, and also it's waterproof, so is a shower chair to boot; and in a box, to be opened in the morning, an electric bath seat thing, that lives in the bath, raises up so you can sit on it and then be gently lowered into the water, with a back rest that you can tip, allowing you to lie in the bath totally supported. I will give it a test-drive tomorrow and report back…

I know we constantly moan about taxes, but come on – we are amazingly privileged to live in a place where this support is available. And all the folk I have met along the way, all of them incredible people – committed, kind, experts. A humbling experience for me.

The lovely Rose was here as well today – giving Clare a manicure, and generally being a Good Egg.

And it seems that the new medications regime is working – Clare is less stoned and very much more on the ball; waking with a smile every time I nudge her to feed her smoothies, or fruit, or pasta. We are still able to goof around – a remarkable achievement from her, and very comforting for me.

Tomorrow we will test-drive the new wheelchair – our mate Fiona will come over and help Clare shower.

And we are thinking of doing a kind of 'Queen's Christmas Message' – as I see I can include audio media on this blog, so we may try and record something of Clare to put on a post in the next few days. Watch this space.

Love to you all.

'Come into the Garden, Maud'

13 AUGUST 2016

I think that was an old Victorian music-hall hit of its day. Just seen – it's actually by Alfred Lord Tennyson. Very posh...

We did a bit of our own 'coming into the garden' this afternoon. I went up the street, mugged my aged mother-in-law and pinched her wheelchair. Managed to get Clare into it, and we had a glorious ten minutes in her back garden, just as the evening sun was dipping behind the big trees. Even so, she tried her best to look like Jackie Onassis – in big sunglasses. So thrilling. A bit of lovely air, watching the bees buzzing through her great swathes of lavender, and getting the scents of all the roses, still in full bloom.

We have test-driven the new commode/shower chair – seems to be a hit. At least for going to the loo. Haven't plucked up courage to have a shower yet. And sad to say, I haven't tried out the new bath seat either.

Clare's friend Grant came over and took her Mini to a garage to get it valued. I had buffed it to a gleaming condition in the morning, desperate to squeeze an extra few pounds from the deal.

And Grant, who is a wizard at all things computery, has sorted out the ability for Clare to dictate emails or Word documents, so we may even be able to post Words from the Horse's Mouth on the next blog.

A great day, all in all. Apart from the fact that England is being stuffed by Pakistan at the cricket. Ah, well. You can't have everything...

Much love to you all.

Washing up

14 AUGUST 2016

All I can remember doing for almost all of the day today was washing up.

And only partly due to the rather lovely soup I made, from French beans, picked from my garden. We are at the time of year when it's beans-a-go-go. Now, don't get me wrong, I love a bean. But there are limits. So a whole pile of beans got thrown with chicken stock and other bits, cooked, whizzed up and made into a gorgeous soup. A small spoon of sour cream, served chilled. Bliss.

Talking of 'serve chilled' – when Clare and I were little, the absolute height of decadence was having fizzy grape juice with Sunday lunch. We were only allowed water at mealtimes normally. The fizz in question was called Shloer – and, as small people, Clare and I misread the serving suggestion on the bottle, and thought it said, 'Best Served Child'.

I may try making French bean ice cream tomorrow, or runner bean cake. I'm sure both are possible...

A quiet day today. I think the trip to the garden yesterday wiped Clare out for the day. Either that, or deep depression that England's cricket team were so badly beaten by Pakistan early this afternoon... I have to say, I will miss listening to *Test Match Special* on the radio – this was the last Test match of the summer. I have had lovely times, sitting in Clare's garden, listening to the commentators leading us through ball-by-ball coverage, and segueing off into all types of conversation (you have to be able to talk at length as cricket is such a slow game) – chats about ancient Greece, how the unit of length known as the metre came into being, rhubarb … I'll have to find some interesting podcasts to keep me going now.

Didn't manage to do much with Clare today. We are focusing on a shower and change of bed-linen tomorrow. But we have had some good talks. Shared thoughts. And the odd gag or two.

And I can tell you, it's one of Life's Great Treats to be able to wake someone, and before they've opened their eyes, see a smile breaking.

Love to you all.

Girding (and washing) of loins …

15 AUGUST 2016

The Internet definition:

Gird (up) your Loins (humorous): to prepare yourself mentally to do something difficult.

This phrase comes from the Bible, where girding up your loins meant to tie up long, loose clothes so that they were more practical when you were working or travelling.

Clare and I mentally girded this morning, and by mid-afternoon were both as prepared as Usain Bolt at the start of his 100 metres. Although we were slightly slower. Using the commode/wheelchair thing, with a couple of towels on the seat to make it a bit softer, we made our gentle way to the shower. And a resounding success. Clare, bless her, totally unfazed by her brother in his underpants (and not even posh Marks & Spencer ones – these, I think, three for £5 at Sainsbury's), washing her hair, helping soap down and rinse off. A quick dash back to the bedroom to change the bottom sheet and lay out towels, before processing back and drying, moisturizing and donning new pyjamas. Huge relief, followed by huge amounts of towel washing and drying – I think we used every bath towel in North London.

And a good dinner of baked cod in tomato, capers and basil, followed by Clare's neighbour's delicious Indian rice pudding.

By 9 p.m., a hospital bed had been delivered, so I will try and get it set up tomorrow. Will manoeuvre Clare onto her sofa in the living room, and then take apart her old bed and put together this new 'whistles and bells' one. I am sure it'll make life so much easier and help with pain, as it tips and folds in various places, has an air-filled mattress, and raises up to make it easier to get out. Hope I can follow the assembly instructions – I'm not very patient with manual-reading – I'll probably build it upside down, so Clare gets regally tipped onto the carpet. Watch this space...

Love to all.

Beer

16 AUGUST 2016

The problem with getting your younger brother to do a manual task after 5 p.m. is that beer enters the equation...

5 p.m. a bit early for the bar to be open, perhaps? I remember when our daughter was a baby, I saved my first beer for when she went to sleep for the night – to start with, 6.30/7 p.m. And did that beer taste great... Then, for some reason, 'Cocktail Hour' slipped. The first beer at bath-time. And then at her 'bottle' time. But 5 p.m. soon became the time – and you can all glean from this that I don't

have a proper job, with proper hours. Although 5 p.m. is sacrosanct. Mostly.

Anyway. The hospital bed needed building, the old bed needed dismantling, and the worker needed help. In the shape of a bottle of Newcastle Brown Ale. One quick slug, and I perched it on the commode/shower chair seat and started attacking Clare's old bed with a monkey wrench. As I took the first pile of timbers away I, of course, knocked over the full bottle, which merrily glugged its foamy contents out all over the carpet. A thorough clean ensued, but there is still a faint whiff of 'pub' about the bedroom…

The bed is in. It raises, tips, angles and can make pretty much any shape you desire. I managed to put it together without bleeding – which is probably a first for me. It also has an electric mattress that keeps inflating and deflating to stop pressure sores, but we don't need that yet. I've hung the control device on a stick taped to the bed frame, so it's easily accessible, although it has ten buttons on it, and Clare needs glasses, so God only knows what shape she'll be in when next I see her…

We had sesame-seeded tuna and garden beans for dinner (yes – beans AGAIN) with our wonderful friend Emma Clarke who had come over to help with some admin.

A last whisky while I type this and hopes for a peaceful night.

Love to all.

Himalaya

17 AUGUST 2016

I spent a rather lovely morning in Clare's garden, lying in the hot sun, reading Michael Palin's travel book *Himalaya*. For those of you not in the know, Palin started out in the comedy world – part of *Monty Python* – then, some years later, found his new niche as a traveller, making films and writing books. I love reading travel books more than anything, and sitting in a garden in North London, I revel in finding myself relocated in the Hindu Kush, the Khyber Pass or Islamabad. But it's the mountains that really draw me. The High Places.

And I suppose I am Sherpa at the moment in Clare's epic mountain climb.

I concentrated on reading and burning my knees this morning, as Clare rested. The afternoon was somewhat busier. A visit from a doctor and nurse from the palliative care crowd, segueing with a lawyer finalizing Clare's will. All very Grown Up. But Clare did beautifully with both professionals.

The upshot – pain meds increased by a significant amount. Let's see how we are over the next days – Clare gets pissed on the sniff of a barmaid's apron, so she will probably be away with the fairies. Which isn't necessarily a bad thing, as she is in pain. And we are still in the time of the caveman when it comes to dealing with pain – it's a sledgehammer approach, unfocused and just sedating. But I don't want to prejudge, so let's see what tomorrow brings...

And, of course, my day would not be complete without more cat-related bemusement. The large grey thing refused to eat his full bowl of food. Continually headbutting me for a whole other full bowl of food. I held fast for most of the day. Finally I gave in – there's a stray cat that hangs around in the garden who gets the food that 'His Highness' doesn't eat, so I scraped out Grably's bowl to put on a plate to put in the garden for our feral friend. No sooner had I scraped it out, than Grably descended on it and ate it all in a one-er. Go figure . . .

Love to all.

Godot

18 AUGUST 2016

Samuel Beckett – one of Ireland's great dramatists – is probably most famous for his play of the early 1950s, *Waiting for Godot*, where the two principal characters spend both halves of the play waiting for someone who never turns up. Just after the play was written, one of the finest and most cutting lines of theatrical critique was penned about the production – summed up as a play 'where nothing happens, twice' . . .

Today nothing happened. But only once.

Clare, both as a result of her new pain meds, and of the huge afternoon yesterday, relaxed all day. Just brief kickings from me to have a smoothie, chicken sandwich (sent back to the kitchen for being 'too dry'), fresh fruit and linguine with bacon and tomato.

She has been, in her own words, relatively pain free, but the blunt instrument of pain medication has just sedated her. Fair enough.

And I was not even able to burn my knees in the garden again today, as it wasn't sunny, so just fussed around with admin. Mostly deleting the hundreds of emails in Clare's inbox, almost all about shopping.

Not even an interesting moment with the cat. It was just one of those days. When nothing happened, but only once...

Love to all.

Oestrogen and Valium

19 AUGUST 2016

It was pointed out to me today that I had missed the very personal connection that Clare has with the play *Waiting for Godot*. Even worse that it was pointed out by her fellow thespian in the production we undertook at school. The protagonists in *Godot* are two tramp-like figures, Estragon and Vladimir. Usually played by men, but in this case, at St Peter's School, York, in I think 1982 (someone I am sure will tell me I am wrong), played by my sister and my then girlfriend, Rose. Thus Estragon and Vladimir became, amongst us thesps, Oestrogen and Valium. It was Rose, and Clare's still top-mate (and mine, obvs), who reminded me of that fact this afternoon.

Circles within circles.

Raining today. Good for the garden. I had to wait in for the delivery of another piece of kit, from the wonderful occupational therapy lot. An above-bed table – you know, the sort they have in hospitals, on wheels. On this we will load all the nonsense Clare needs to hand at night, as she can't reach over to her bedside table very easily. Useful for cards as well.

The table is built now and in place. Although, rather annoyingly, it only stretches over half the width of the bed. No good for billiards, then. I will 'pimp' it up before bedtime, working out where everything needs to be, and with my handy roll of gaffer tape to make sure nothing moves in the night.

Clare is worried about 'night starvation'. I don't know how many of you know about the malted drink Horlicks – it's basically malty powder that you add hot milk to. Allegedly a sleep aid, and in the early 1930s it marketed itself on combating 'night starvation' – God knows how we all get through the night without it... To combat Clare's worries, tonight, on her new above-bed table, will be a veritable banquet of fresh fruit salad, some tinned rice pudding (which she will only eat cold. Never hot) and a banana – pre-nicked at the end, for ease of opening. If that doesn't work, I tell her, tomorrow it will be a boar and a flagon of mead.

Right. Time for teeth-brushing and a trip to the loo. Then the symphony of medications. All written down on a piece of paper in the meds drawer, so I don't go 'off-piste'. Would hate to get her stoned again...

Love to all.

NHS DIY

20 AUGUST 2016

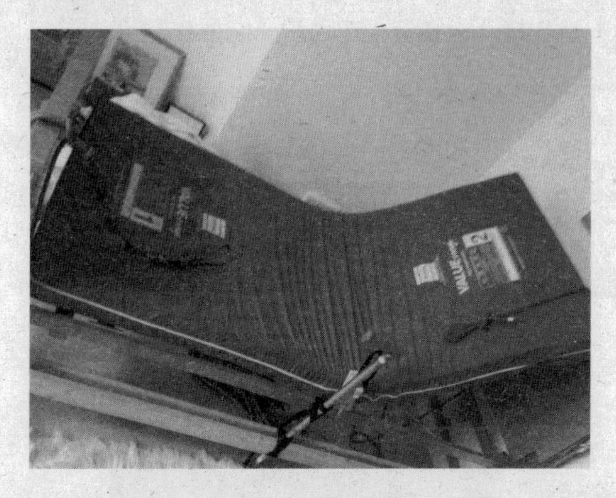

Steph has asked for me to include a photo of how I can 'pimp up', with my do-it-yourself skills, whatever our National Health Service throws at me. The photo is actually from last summer, when I nicked my mum-in-law's bed for Clare – a shackled walking stick (attached to two timber bearers I had affixed to the bed's base), and my climbing rope, knotted at intervals to help Clare pull herself up to sitting, or back along the bed to lie down. This was when she'd just been diagnosed, and I'm afraid that climbing ropes would not be much use to her now. Although this system is presently being used by my mum-in-law, very successfully. As life always likes to keep you on your toes, my mum-in-law was diagnosed with Parkinson's a week or so ago. My suggestion was to put her and Clare in a double bed together, top-to-toe, so that every once in a while they could push their control buttons, raise themselves, and have a chat (probably about the shoddy standard of nursing they are subject to . . .).

This photo is one I found recently – of the two of us in the late 1960s. I'm the one on the right. Clare looking embarrassed as she's probably just realized she's forgotten to put any trousers on . . . And you can probably tell that our mum cut our hair.

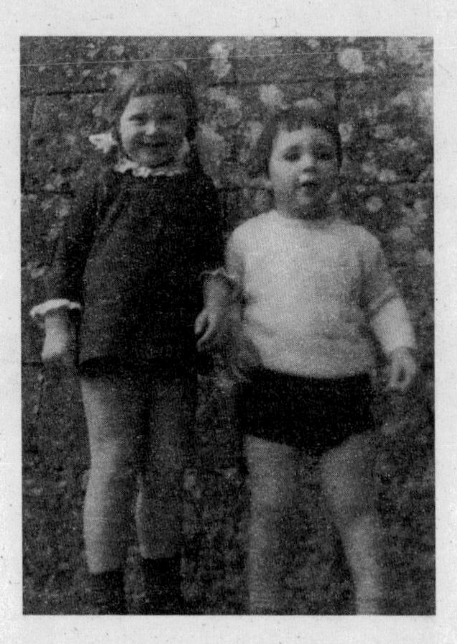

Clare managed to get through last night without starvation – actually didn't really touch anything, but I'll continue to make sure there are lovely titbits on offer (for those of you in the US, confused at this, please read 'tidbits' – whatever a tidbit is . . .).

I really should learn the magician's trick of being able to pull away a tablecloth at speed, leaving everything still in place on the table. On taking Clare to the loo this afternoon, I went into hyper-drive – attempting a whole bed-linen change – I feel fairly confident that I could be in the pit-stop team on Formula 1 racing now. Almost managed it in the time allotted to empty a bladder. And a change of pyjamas to boot. We were planning on a shower, but are lightly pencilling that for tomorrow afternoon – can't have too much excitement in one day, and fresh linen should be enough of an achievement.

That's what is clear at this time – celebrate the small things, the small moments. I think it's probably a Buddhist thing (or some New Age nonsense, more likely) that if you find yourself with matching socks as you leave the house in the morning, that is a cause for celebration. And I couldn't agree more. If the rest of the day is spent finding the cure for cancer, or brokering World Peace, then that's a bonus.

And there are gems, there are tiny powerful moments, if we just make ourselves available to witness and mark them. They are there, every day, all around us.

Here Endeth the Sermon.

Love to all.

Khyber Pass

21 AUGUST 2016

Clare's flat is on a hill. The name of the street has 'Hill' in it – it's that sort of incline. London is famous for its subsoil – 'London Clay' – thick, green-grey heavy clay, that I'm sure you could turn into pottery. Clay reacts to groundwater and drought in a fairly excessive fashion: swelling, shrinking, cracking... Thus three-storey houses built on a hill, on clay, tend to want to relocate the way gravity takes them. Downwards. (Not good for property prices, as the posher houses are at the top of the hill, but I digress...) When Clare bought her flat, we discovered that her bedroom floor had a difference in height of two or three inches between the walls, due to the subsidence over the years. Now, you can either throw money at the issue – take up the floor, pack out the joists, and re-lay the now-levelled floor. Or, if you've spent all the money you have in the world (and quite a bit more) purchasing your dream property, you call your brother. Who calls a mate. Between us, we nailed all sorts of various thicknesses of wood onto the heavily inclined floor, and laid on top of them eight-foot-by-four-foot sheets of plywood. Thus making a levelled floor for Clare – hurrah. But a levelled floor that was a good inch higher than the rest of the flooring in her house. Not to worry – a lovely carpet was laid on the plywood and a lovely oak sill, chamfered (i.e. – angled) made the underfoot portal between hallway and bedroom. Gorgeous.

Until you have to start having to negotiate the change in level with the commode/wheelchair. Not a normal wheelchair with bicycle tyres and suspension: an unforgiving, small-solid-wheeled utilitarian contraption, where Clare feels every tiny jolt and bang. So, manoeuvring over this 'Khyber Pass' has been something of a pain – pulling the front wheels of the chair to the sill, lifting the whole front of the chair, and repositioning the wheels on the other side, to be repeated with the back wheels. And in the wee small hours of the night, on the way to the loo, fraught with anxiety – mostly on my part – as the last thing I want to do is to cause any pain.

So, I took out this lovely sill. Found a couple of thin pieces of wood in Clare's wood store, and gaffer-taped them to the change in level. And it works like a dream.

We were able to glide over the junction this afternoon, and Clare spent a good hour on her sofa, looking out of the patio doors to the garden beyond; me showing her various emails from the last days (not the shopping ones) and her being able to have a proper change of scene.

Took it out of her, though, and the rest of the day has been spent in bed. Fair enough. We expanded horizons, and then retrenched.

Didn't manage a shower. But tomorrow is another day...

Love to all.

A 'water stripe'

22 AUGUST 2016

What is a 'water stripe'?

This was requested by Clare at some point in the wee small hours of last night. She had recently had enormous amounts of pain meds exploded into her system, and was pretty stoned. I had recently been dragged out of deep sleep to facilitate whatever it was she needed. And we found ourselves at an impasse. A water stripe... a water stripe... aaaah, of course: a straw. Clare drinks her water out of the glass with a stripy straw. We got there in the end: a multi-dimensional game of charades, word association and theatre games. Similar to the fun we all had (those of us who are parents, anyway) with our small children when they tried to explain a word they don't know with words they did. Actually, German is a rather good language for this – if you don't know the word, you can probably make it up with a couple of words you do know. They are great fans of what is known, I believe, as a 'compound noun' – just mash words together to make a new one. We do it in English as well – 'wristwatch' in German is '*Armbanduhr*', basically a 'bracelet-clock'. Graceful. Less graceful is this one – a sixty-three-letter compound noun, allegedly the longest word in German. Ready?

Rindfleischetikettierungsüberwachungsaufgabenübertragungsgesetz.

The word, which means 'the law concerning the delegation of duties for the supervision of cattle marking and the labelling of beef', was introduced in 1999. It was given the abbreviation *RkReÜAÜG*, thankfully. Although try pronouncing that.

I am so glad that Clare isn't concerned with labelling-of-beef issues at 3 a.m...

After a rather difficult night, with awakenings every couple of hours, I needed to get out of the flat for a moment this morning, so I dragged the mother-in-law's helper down the street, to 'hold the fort' while I zoomed around on the bike, picking up various prescriptions and bits of shopping. And was finally able to finish making my batch of damson jam that I've been preparing over the last days: gathering the fruit; stoning the fruit; buying the sugar; sterilizing the jars... nine pounds of jam, all jarred up this morning. An honouring of the ancient damson tree in our garden.

Shebo, our wonderful Macmillan nurse, popped by at lunchtime to check that all was well. We are going to try a new way of getting through nights without pain and thus regular waking – an injection, just before bed, of a drug that Clare takes at the moment in pill form. A district nurse will come when we wish and give Clare the injection. I think we can start this regime tomorrow at bedtime. And hopefully quiet nights will ensue.

When my daughter Gaia was in the last months of her primary school, aged eleven (2011), and had already passed the exam to get into 'Big School', we took her out of school and round the world for just under five months: Borneo, Australia, Brazil, and then Ecuador and the Galapagos, where Clare joined us. Who knew that my sister, this fantastically cultured urbanite, would love the extremes of the Amazonian rainforest as much as she did? I was in awe of her. The top photo is way, way up in the primary forest canopy, on a reasonably rickety platform, searching for macaws; the bottom one is the two of us, I think looking at a sloth, on a tiny tributary of the Amazon. She was a wonderful, intrepid, fearless explorer. And still is. And I am still in awe.

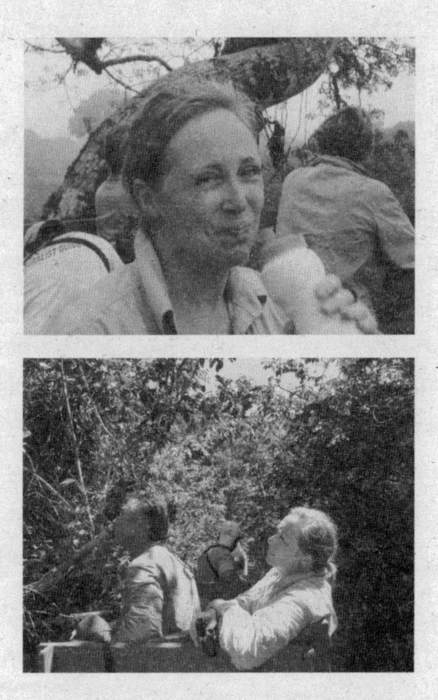

Just settled her down for the night. Wish us luck.

Love to all.

Ice lollies on the couch

23 AUGUST 2016

Phew, what a scorcher...

Hot, hot, hot today.

Unfortunately, we had another rather bumpy night last night. Although the start of my nocturnal wakenings was due to the crying baby in the flat above me. Bless it. I hope I got my own back at around 3 a.m., when Clare requested a fruit smoothie, so I gleefully ran the decibel-busting NutriBullet for a good few seconds more than was actually required. Childish of me, I know. But you have to score the points where you can. And a fifty-year-old man versus a baby??? It's an open goal...

I spent the morning in the Himalayas with Michael Palin in Clare's garden, gently re-burning my knees, but by lunchtime the request came through from the bedroom for a 'change of scene'. Now that Clare has the posh 'whistles-and-bells' hospital bed, her old inflating pillow-raiser has been relegated to the basement. But a few minutes and a few yards of string later, and the old pillow-raiser found itself tied on the end of the couch. Clare could therefore lie at whatever angle she wanted – relaxing, looking at the garden, or, as transpired early afternoon, sitting and working her way, very professionally, through a strawberries-and-cream ice lolly. Glorious to behold.

The freezer is now filled with various assortments of lolly – I hope I have covered whatever takes her fancy in the coming days. I did have to throw a few out that I'd found earlier – notably a 'Mojito Poptail', which had, in big letters underneath: 'Contains Alcohol'...

probably not the iced-treat-of-choice for someone with as many opiates in her system as my sister.

The district nurses turned up this evening, but after seeing Clare, decided against giving her the big shot of painkillers. As she was pretty relaxed already, they were anxious that knocking her out for the night wasn't necessarily the best course of action. Fair enough. So, let's hope for a calm baby upstairs, and a calm sister down the hall.

Love to all.

Scrooge

24 AUGUST 2016

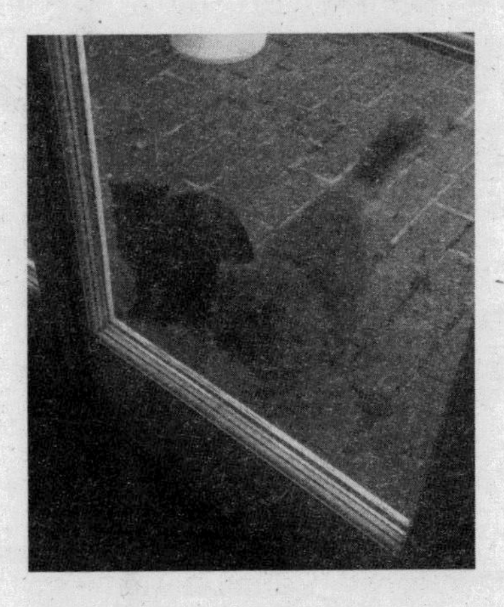

This is the sight that greeted me this morning, on shuffling my way to the kitchen to make Clare's breakfast smoothie: two very middle-class, very well-fed felines on a balmy summer's morn, giving their best Bob Cratchit and Tiny Tim, freezing and starving in a cold Dickensian winter…

I left them outside. I'm that kind of guy.

Another hot day today. Not a lot of movement from the sis, but I've lost count of the smoothies she's consumed – very heartening, as I use a base of a prescription drink called Ensure that has all the various vitamins, minerals, etc., in it you need, but, as it's calorie-rich, it's wildly sweet – so, mixed in with that and whizzed up, a combination of raspberries, blueberries, galia melon, nectarine, banana, apple and a dash of lemon juice. Very scrummy.

I know we live in a time when we can get everything we want whenever we want. And, being an old fart, sometimes that saddens me. I remember the wild excitement of spending summers with my German cousins and coming back to the UK with a jar of Nutella (for those of you not in the know, a chocolate/hazelnut spread, to top toast, ice cream, or whatever); the great joy of midsummer, just at the moment of the Wimbledon tennis championships – the first strawberries. Amazing. Now I can buy Nutella not 100 metres from where I'm typing this, in the same store that sells strawberries year-round. But... and there is a point to this rant... the fruits we are eating now, in our summer, the fruits I am whizzing up for Clare's smoothies: berries, peaches, nectarines, are all so wonderfully tasty – because they are in season, locally. Not brought, semi-ripe and chilled, halfway across the world by plane, but picked when ripe and eaten within moments. And the taste is the taste of pure, juicy, ripe summer. I tried to instill in my daughter, Gaia, the idea of eating seasonally – and I started to do this by planting vegetables in our garden in London – so that she knows not only where the various fruits and vegetables come from, but when they are pickable. I know I banged on a few posts ago about the glut of beans emanating from my garden at this time, but I still get a thrill from picking a bean that I have grown from a bean, pressed into compost in a pot, back in March.

I'm wittering now. Apologies. This is what comes from days with nobody to talk to. Apart from brief exchanges with Clare, which are either about the domestic, or slightly drug-fuelled. I'm having my first beer of the evening – it's nearly 6 p.m. – maybe the heat and the alcohol are getting to me...

I just checked my weather app – according to them at 6 p.m. in London it is 91 degrees (that's 33 Celsius) – I must have sunstroke.

Love to you all.

Big game hunter

25 AUGUST 2016

I have been known to spend an entire night, in various bedrooms over the world, searching out and attempting to eviscerate a lone mosquito. The last of the Big Game Hunters. I found myself doing so again last night. As my head hit the pillow, the ominous high-pitched whine started. I realized – as I had just dispatched mosquito number four, by balancing myself on Clare's old bedhead, which is now shoved up against the wall in the room where I am sleeping, and lunging upwards, wobbling dramatically, with a rather flimsy green plastic fly swat – that I should probably stop. I am someone who can bleed profusely as a result of unwrapping a birthday present, and Clare really doesn't need a carer with more fractures than her...

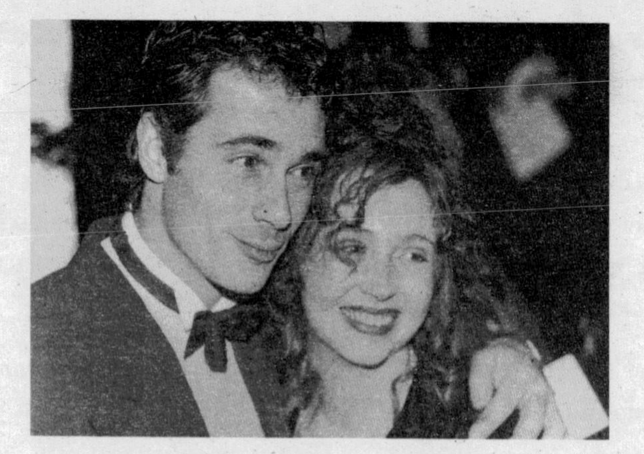

I was asked to include more photos – so here's one I just found in Clare's study. The two of us at the premiere party of *Sense and Sensibility*, back in 1996. I am in a borrowed suit, but very much own the pout. Clare is sporting an eighties' Cyndi Lauper hairstyle for some reason…

A better night last night. A calmer Clare and a sharper brother – I knew exactly what was meant at around 4 a.m., when Clare asked for 'fat-bottomed water' – sparkling water, natch.

Busy morning – my weekly drug inventory, sorting new meds to be prescribed; finally washing the shorts I have been wearing non-stop for a month (a better option than the two others I was toying with: either boiling them up to make soup, or ceremoniously throwing them on a pyre in the back garden). Endless emails, both mine and Clare's; shouting at a poor girl from Visa (actually, not shouting, but being 'disappointed', which is much scarier) and fielding dozens of phone calls. Bless all of you who read the last blog about me not having anyone to talk to during the days – I was inundated with calls today. But you misunderstand me – I wasn't looking for pity – I don't like talking: just ask the wife…

Talking of the wife – has anyone seen her recently? She and Gaia have been in the far north of the Canadian Arctic on a Greenpeace mission for the last couple of weeks. I think they've been tweeting, or Facebooking, or something, about it. I have no idea, as I don't do either, but see if you can see what they've been up to.

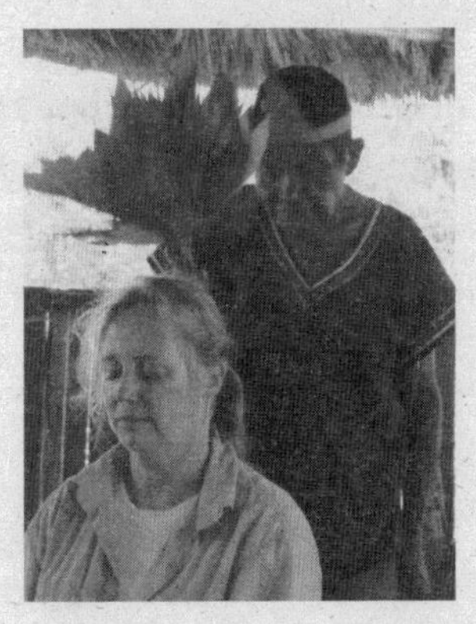

More photos for you image-hungry crazy-cats. Ecuador, again, June 2011, with Clare going through a shamanic ritual, in a tiny village in the rainforest. That worked, then . . .

Iceland. November 2013. Clare was desperate to see the Northern Lights – so, as a celebration of the end of the chemotherapy for her

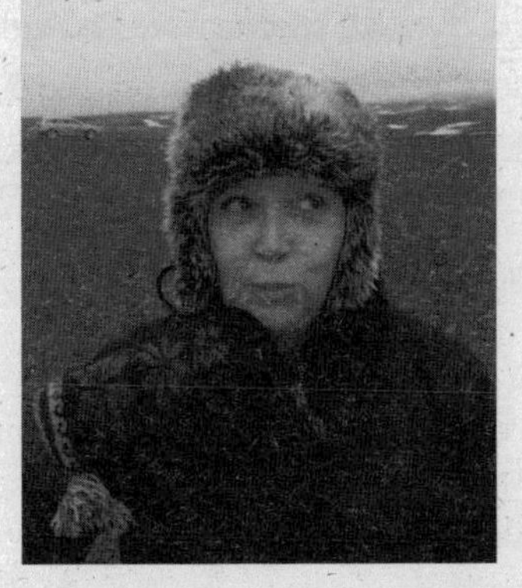

Looking coy on a lava field. I don't really know what else you can do on a lava field

breast cancer, a 'thank you' to her wonderful chum Esther, who had come over from Australia to live with her for the months of treatment, and a way of getting Gaia out of school for a few days, we all went off to Iceland. And we got to see the aurora borealis (the posh name for the Northern Lights) – for about thirty seconds at 2 a.m. on a freezing hillside...

It's 7.30 p.m. now. I'm drinking a bottle of beer called Naked Ladies. Rather lovely, and making me feel slightly naughty – until I see that it was brewed in Twickenham: where the English National Rugby stadium is. Not that sexy, then...

Better get the sis ready for bed. Wish us luck.

Love to all.

Spa day

26 AUGUST 2016

One of the positive things about getting older, if by older you also mean a little wiser, is that you get to know your limits.

This is the great game played out from almost the first proper thoughts of a child, through adolescence and upwards – 'What are my limits?' 'What is possible?' – and we spend our formative years pushing against what is put in our way to limit us; and through that pushing, we see where our power lies, and what we can achieve (or at least get away with...).

And over the fifty years of life that I have thus far lived, one thing, above others, has become crystal clear to me: I am about as far away from being an esthetician as is humanly possible... (and no, I had no idea there was a word for it – look it up...) Basically – I'm not a Spa Guy.

We had got to the stage where Clare needed a wash. And the thought of her brother in his cheap underpants wheeling her into a lukewarm shower just didn't do it for her.

It's been hot, hot, hot for days now. And even with fans, and loose bedcovers, Clare has – now, what is the word? Horses sweat, men perspire, ladies glow – anyway, she has been glowing like a 100-watt light bulb. And needed help.

To the rescue came the 'Spa Girls' – in the shape of her old chums Fiona, Phillipa and Rose. As I was doing 'boy things' (cycling around to pick up meds and new pyjamas), the girls sprang into action, and bathed, lotioned and generally primped my sister – all within the confines of her bed. And I returned, a sweaty, cyclist mess, to a fragrant, clean and relaxed sibling. How lovely...

We also had a visit from a doctor and the amazing Shebo, our nurse – mainly to calm me down with various telephone numbers, as we are hitting a three-day holiday now, and thus our usual support team will not be around. Monday is a bank holiday: lovely for 'the Workers', but not so good if you need help. But I have been assured that help will always be at hand, and will say a little prayer to the Universe that help will not be required.

Clare has been good today. Sleeping mostly, but not in pain, and with no anxiety. Let's all hope that this continues – so, whatever you believe, whoever you think has the power, just say a few words for a peaceful few days for our Clare.

And love to you all. And if you're in the UK reading this, have a great bank holiday weekend.

All quiet on the north-west London front

27 AUGUST 2016

Anyone remember the book *All Quiet on the Western Front* written by Erich Maria Remarque, a German veteran of the terrible battles of the Western Front in the First World War? I think it was on the English syllabus when I was at school. And I remember reading it with a little more interest than I showed in most of the books I was forced to read at school, as my (and thus Clare's) maternal grandfather fought on the Western Front. For the Germans. Or for the Prussians, as I think he would have liked them to have been called.

Clare and I had a good conversation about all of this a few weeks ago. About the fabulous random nature of our appearance on this earth – a grandmother from Croatia, a grandfather from Transylvania (both of them officially 'Hungarian' at that time – with the huge Austro-Hungarian empire straddling all under it), and another grandmother and grandfather from the north of England. Eva and Emil begat our mother in Paris; and Doris and Horace (I kid you not) begat our father in, I believe, Redcar. At least, that's where he was born. And through all sorts of quirks of fate, our mum and dad found themselves at university together in Newcastle.

We are all products of such 'accidents of birth' – to have happened to have been born where we were, when we were, parented by our parents. All just accidents.

And that is why I find it so hard to understand Nationalism, or Racism – the fear of 'the Other', as we are all products of incredible probabilities stacked against any of us ever turning up. And any of us could have been born anywhere, at any time, any colour, to any couple . . .

This is a very long-winded way of me saying that it is all quiet here. We had a reasonably good night – only two wakings, and the day has been calm. Hot and muggy still, so I kick the sis every hour or so and make sure she's hydrating. Lots of smoothies, lots of fizzy water (fat-bottomed water, for those of you who are paying attention) with elderflower cordial; the fan is on, a loose sheet on the bed, and from time to time, a nice cold flannel on the forehead.

And a bit more about 'accidents' – Clare's brother (me) chanced to meet a half-Scottish, half-English woman, and a niece was produced:

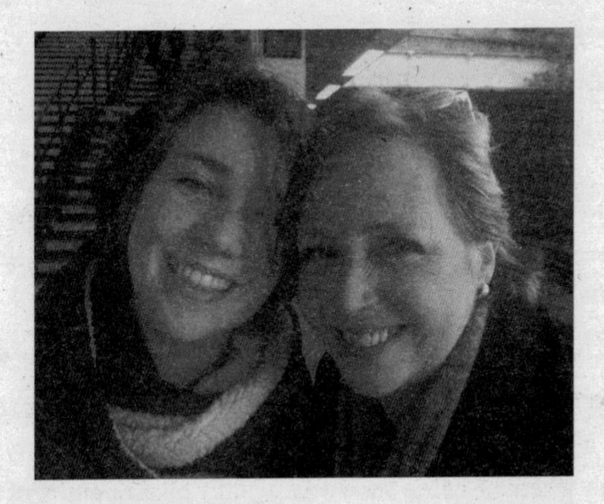

And, rather naughtily of me, but that's what little brothers are for: a photo from a couple of years ago, when her hair was starting to grow back in after the chemotherapy. Just to show that you can't escape your genes: Clare with a photo of the baby Clare – remarkable similarity, don't you think???

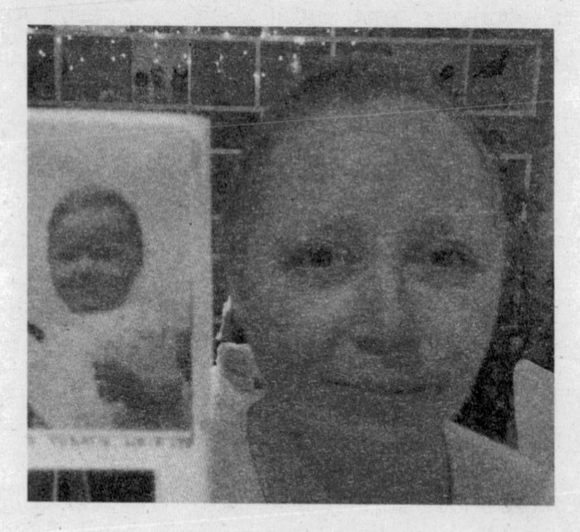

Love to all.

First Law of Thermodynamics

28 AUGUST 2016

As far as I understand it, the First Law of Thermodynamics says that energy cannot be created or destroyed – merely transformed from one form to another.

I started musing on this earlier today, when I witnessed Grably the cat (and apologies for those of you eating whilst reading this...) having a huge poo in his litter box and proceeding directly to his food tray where he gulped down an equally huge quantity of food – energy merely transformed from one form to another...

Or maybe I am slightly confused by thermodynamics.

(This, of course, is not to be confused with the Law of Beer-o-dynamics, which states that the amount of time spent drinking beer without going to the toilet equals the amount of time then spent going to the toilet without drinking beer.)

Last week I watched a series of documentaries about the universe – every atom in everything we can see, everywhere, all came from the Big Bang, and has just been circulating in various forms ever since.

Atoms in my body, today, may once have been in a tree in Australia, a fish in the Bay of Bengal, a glacier in the Arctic, in Attila the Hun's toenail or Moses' spleen (that wasn't in the documentary, by the way. This is just me being random).

I love this thought. Nothing is created nor destroyed – just keeps, eternally, passing through the universe, stopping for a while and then moving on.

And that thought soothes me, witnessing what is happening to my sister.

A gloriously calm night last night. I woke, unbidden, looked at the clock: 4 a.m. Thought I'd better go and check on the sis, wandered into her room and was greeted by an 'Oh, how lovely to see you.' (It was like she was channelling the Queen at a garden party.) 'Lovely to see you, too,' I replied. (See how polite we Brits are??) She, of course, needed many things, but had just not quite got around to summoning me by the bell. After a loo stop, a full glass of smoothie, a fresh one put on her table and a couple of pills, I wandered off to bed again. Next wake 9.30 a.m. Wow. Looked in on Herself and saw her bed sheet splattered with fruity shrapnel from her smoothie drinking, and (so you all know that the 'old Clare' is still very much present) – she just looked at me, wryly, and said, 'Sorry – all a bit *Texas Chainsaw Massacre*...'

Most of today she has been in a deep sleep. I have tried my usual hand stroking and gentle calling to wake her, but to no avail. So I just left her, checking in every wee while. Woke her, finally, at about 4 p.m., and she was cross that so much of the day had gone to waste. Thus we had more smoothies, did a spot of cleansing and moisturizing, and chewed the fat, for some considerable time, about all sorts of things – films, friends, the weather, the news, how tasty the smoothie was. I told her I'd been banging on in the blog about 'seasonality' of fruit and veg, and she reminded me that when we were kids – probably no older than ten or twelve – in late October at our cottage in Northumberland (far north of England), we would help with the potato harvest. The tractor would go in front of us, with some grubbing-up machine at the back, and we would walk behind, with sacks, and pick the potatoes out of the freezing, wet, clodded earth. Absolutely back-breaking. But we got 50p an hour, so by the end of the weekend, had somewhere north of £5. Riches! (We worked out that our pocket money at the time was probably around 20p a week.) And a great perk of doing this job was that the farmer allowed us to have a turnip from a big pile in his field (this is sounding terribly *Blackadder*, but I promise it's true) that we could take home and hollow out as a Halloween lantern (this in the days before we had even heard of pumpkins). I always chose the biggest one, which was thus the toughest one to hollow out – using a teaspoon, as you couldn't give a child like me a knife (you still really shouldn't). I don't know if anyone out there has ever tried to hollow out a turnip with a teaspoon, but it makes Sisyphus's task look like a stroll in the park...

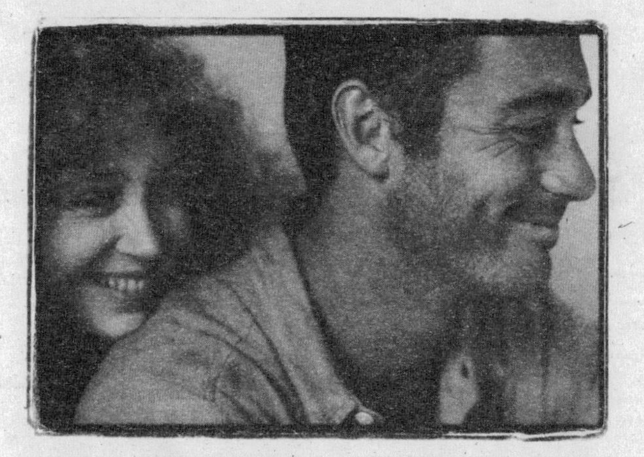

Couldn't find a photo of the two of us at that age, so here's one probably ten or so years later (that I think our pal Rose took) – with the two of us obviously still giddy from our potato-picking earnings.

Love to all.

Problem-solving

29 AUGUST 2016

Clare and I are both big problem-solvers. I don't mean sudoku, or crosswords (although I do love a cryptic crossword), but actual in-front-of-your-eyes problems.

What she is going through now throws up an almost constant stream of new problems. Things as simple as drinking: the numbness on the right side of her face means she can't really close that side of her mouth now, so drinking with a straw can be problematic – more air coming in at the corner of her mouth, than suction up the straw. So, over the past days, we have tried out various combinations of drinking appliances (just stopping short of a watering can). She will suggest something, we'll 'road-test' it. It'll work for a day or two, and then we'll have to rethink.

And Clare will almost always have a suggestion.

We have, I feel, found a wonderful partnership. And more than anything, I have cherished her constant focus on trying to find solutions. At the same time, allowing me to facilitate what she has come up with. It is a hard thing to do, to accept help. It is so much easier to give.

Clare has always been a great one for an agenda, for planning, for schedules, lists, objectives, timescales. Even when we were young children – and fortunate enough to have our own space: a 'playroom' in our house, that opened onto a big lawn and garden. Not surprisingly, all the local kids would congregate at ours, slightly at a loose end, as kids often are. Within seconds, Clare would have organized a game, a dressing-up adventure, a puppet show. Later on, at sixteen, she came to the school I'd been at for most of my time – a boys' school, that had girls join in the Sixth Form. Before the end of her first term there, she was known as 'Clipboard Clare' – always the organizer.

And here we differ. I've always found it hard to put things into a diary. I feel trapped by the idea of a mapped-out, scheduled, fixed time ahead. An old girlfriend threatened to leave me if I didn't get a Filofax (she left me even after I got one...) as I was always a bit too woolly about future plans.

This is something which is very apparent in Clare now – there is no 'shape' to things, no agenda, no diary. Often, when I raise her from a deep sleep, she will ask me about appointments, and times. She needs to know constantly what time it is, what day it is – I told her today was Monday, and she murmured that she really had to write it down.

So we are both confronting things new – she has no agenda, and I am required to plan ahead (with regard to making sure we have enough meds); keep focused on timing (hydrating, feeding, giving meds), and actually having to keep the place tidy (the bits she sees, anyway).

But I'll never be 'Clipboard Greg'...

Love to all.

Military precision

30 AUGUST 2016

Clare has taken to saluting me. I am, of course, flattered. But slightly worried that she's using her left arm in the salutation (as her right one has a 30-centimetre metal pin in it, and pathologic fractures). I just checked on the Internet, and luckily there is a clause about using the wrong arm:

> *'... the left hand can be used when it is the only possible way to salute, i.e. broken arm. But, even though this is acceptable it is usually never done, at least in the Marine Corps.'*

So now we all know...

I suppose this is a postscript to yesterday's blog, about us problem-solving together; about trying to find order, rhythm, ease and, just creeping in from time to time, a bit of levity. I may run this particular sanitorium with military precision, but can still be openly mocked by my sis.

As I went off for a bit of 'emotional housekeeping' this afternoon (my weekly trip to my therapist), Clare got a bit of 'physical housekeeping', in the form of another spa. A lovely cleanse, lotions, new sheets and new outfit, thanks to Philly and Rose.

Clare cannot stop herself from being the Hostess – she will always enquire after everyone else in the room (I was met at 3 a.m. by a 'How *are* you – did you sleep well?'), will always need to know that everyone is being well looked after. Thus, even a spa is taxing – and by the time I got back at 5ish, Clare was lying exhausted on the sofa. Too tired to stand. But as her energy is so finite now, I can think of no better use of whatever reserves she has than just to have a small nugget of normality – old chums, a bit of chat, a cup of tea and a facial.

The whole standing issue is a new problem that we'll have to find a solution for (sorry for ending a sentence with a preposition...). Without her being able to swing her legs out of bed, stand, pirouette and get onto the wheelchair/commode thing, we won't be able to go to the loo. We faced this first thing this morning, but approached it in a calm, problem-solving manner: a big glass of energy-filled smoothie, a half-hour snooze, and 'ker-pow' – standing, and thus going to the loo was (apologies for the vulgar pun) 'a piece of piss'...

But thank goodness – the answer to all our problems landed on our doormat today:

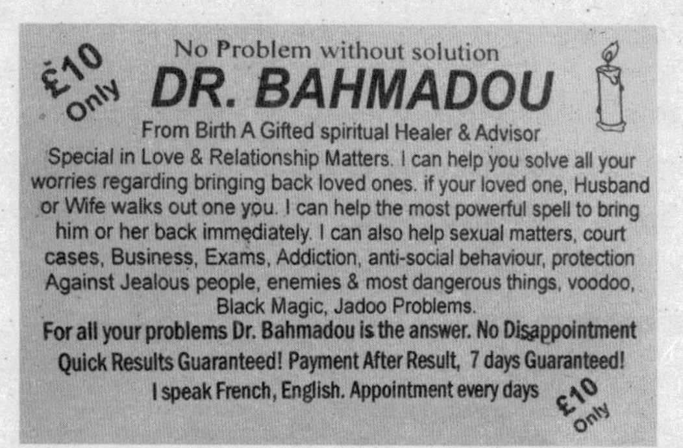

I'm thinking of giving him a call – if nothing else, the £10 payment *after* results seems rather hopeful, although he may ask for the money upfront in Clare's case.

Love to all.

Metoclopramide

31 AUGUST 2016

Metoclopramide. OxyNorm. OxyContin. Duloxetine. Ranitidine. Dexamethasone...

Who came up with these polysyllabic names? (Chemists, I suppose.) How are we mere mortals supposed to remember them, what dose, and what they're for? Luckily I have a crib sheet in the meds drawer with doses, and every packet is written on, by me, in big red letters – 'anti-nausea', 'anti-anxiety', 'stomach-protector', etc.

Some time ago, Clare and I started calling various of the meds by nicknames – thus Effentora (a crazy painkiller in pill form, dissolving in the mouth, acting like an injection – almost instantaneous relief) became 'Nora Ephron' (screenwriter of such things as *When Harry Met Sally* and *You've Got Mail*, and who we both thought spelled her name Effron – hence our terribly witty gag. But we were wrong...). So our shorthand when in pain would be asking for a 'Nora'. If only in a little pain, I'd halve the pill – that was a 'Zac' (Zac Efron – young heart-throb actor of *High School Musical*, etc. – God, we're funny...).

This worked well, until in moments of delirium, when we'd both get terribly confused by our shorthand. So it's Effentora, pure and simple, now.

This is a pill that you only really need when you're in great pain. So, naturally, getting the pill out of its covering shouldn't be easy in any way. It is one of the most difficult endeavours I've ever undertaken. No 'blister pack' for this puppy – oh no, that would be too straightforward: a hard plastic carapace with an incredibly sticky foil-backed covering that I have to prise apart with tweezers, often crumbling the delicate pill in the process...

Lorazepam – an anti-anxiety pill – was always small, oblong and blue. Hence known by the two of us as a 'Bluey'. Until a recent prescription, when it appeared in round and white form – exactly like the Effentora pills. At night I put a little bowl on Clare's over-bed table with some halved Effentoras ('Zacs'), next to which lies a blister strip of Lorazepam, to which is affixed a sticky label with a huge black 'L' written on it: just so she doesn't get confused in the night between the two meds that she can self-prescribe. Now, though, the *new* prescription of Lorazepam is back to the small, blue, oblong pills again... Even I'm confused.

Clare had her nails done this afternoon by the lovely Emma and Philly, whilst I stole myself up the road to my place for a most-overdue shower. Our glorious nurse, Shebo, came over and we have worked on little achievable goals – especially being able to stand with ease. So, tomorrow, Clare and I are going to try a bit of bed physiotherapy: gentle movements that will help her upper legs, thus facilitating standing and sitting. Her core strength is still great: she can do sit-ups like an Olympic gymnast. One with cancer, anyway.

It's all about Little Victories: drinking a glass of smoothie (and without the *Texas Chainsaw Massacre* effect); getting out of bed and onto the wheelchair; managing to take the plethora of polysyllabic pills without choking; successful teeth-brushing. All things marked and celebrated. All we have now – all any of us has ever had, if truth be told – are the Little Victories.

Love to all.

'Presenter One'

1 SEPTEMBER 2016

There has been a dearth of photos in the last few blogs, which I will set right a bit further down this page. I found another couple of shots of me and Clare from an album in my study. And a strange thought struck me as I copied them. Clare, in every photo I can find, is on my right (and thus on the left in the photo).

And I remembered a bit of an argument that blew up in the media a few months ago, about the positioning of male and female presenters on sofas on TV programmes – that the male presenter is always on the left (as we view it), and this was seen as a sort of 'Sofa Sexism'. I did some digging, and found:

> *'the left seat (as seen by viewers) on the sofa is said to denote seniority, termed "Presenter One" by programme makers.'*

Clare, always on my right: by engineering, by luck, or more probably the universe telling everyone that in our pairing, she is very much 'Presenter One'.

(The only photo I found that differed was from the *Sense and Sensibility* party, where I assume we were wrangled by a photographer – as, probably for the only time in our relationship, I was 'Presenter One' that evening…)

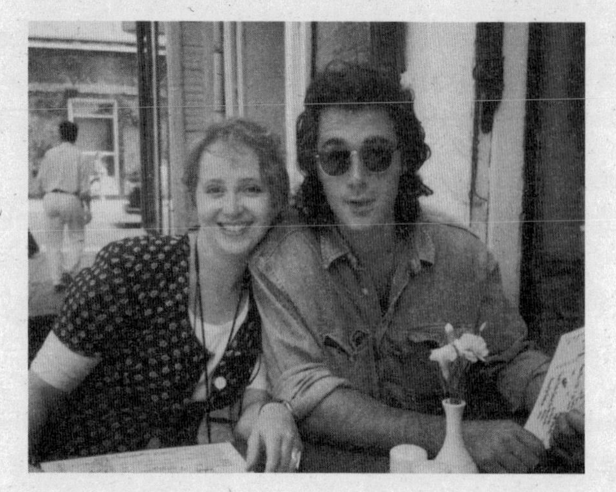

See??

This, I think, was taken in Venice. Probably when we went Interrailing (a month's train pass in Europe for young people) back in the mid-1980s (can't you tell by my hair???).

And this – taken in a local park – I assume pre-children, as my hair is yet to turn white. My silly little beard was for a film – honest.

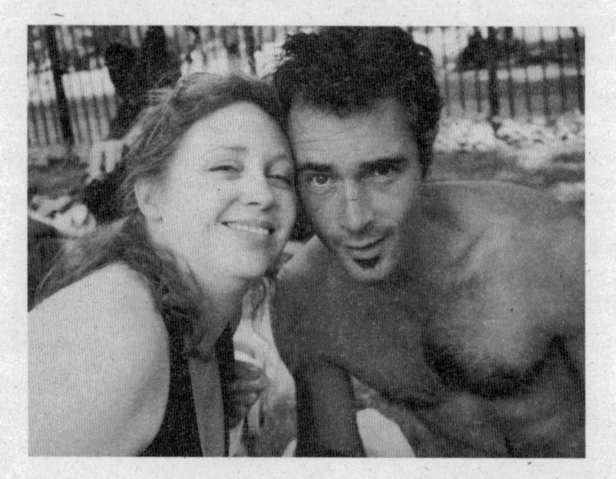

After a reasonably bumpy night last night (bell-ringing at 1, 3 and 5 a.m.), a quiet day today. Punctuated only by the screaming of the baby, and the endless sprinting of the toddler upstairs.

I managed some time in the September sun in the garden. Now reading Bruce Chatwin's *In Patagonia* – a book I first read probably thirty years ago. So beautifully written, and I am with him every step of his journey through that wild and desolate South American landscape. Lost in his words until snapped out of my reverie by a crash and thump – drag my eyes from the book to watch a squirrel attempting to cram a horse chestnut into its mouth in the tree above. (Goodness me – I just Googled it and to my amazement found it is in the lychee family. Who knew?)

The horse chestnut, at this time of year, when I was a small lad, was so incredibly exciting, as its fruits gave you 'conkers' (often not 'giving', but forced to drop them as a consequence of having sticks thrown up into the canopy to dislodge the prize) – according to Wikipedia:

> *'Conkers is a traditional children's game in Britain and Ireland played using the seeds of horse chestnut trees… The game is played by two players, each with a conker threaded onto a piece of string: they take turns striking each other's conker until one breaks.'*

We would soak our conkers in vinegar, or bake them in the oven (allegedly both things strengthened them), bored holes in them and threaded string through. Kept in a bag that would be your constant companion at school in the weeks ahead. If you were victorious in the battle, your conker became a 'One-er', then a 'Two-er'… more victories, more numbers – possibly reaching the heady heights of many tens.

Again, I am showing what an old fart I am, but the game isn't played any more. And this time of the year fills me with a gentle sadness, when I pick up endless beautiful conkers from the ground under the trees, just left to rot…

Fi came over this afternoon to do a bit more spa-work on Clare. Tuesday had been body, yesterday nails and today was going to be hair. I went to the local pharmacy and had a funny few minutes there with the pharmacist – both of us men, him bald, trying to figure out what 'dry shampoo' is… I eventually brought back two options: a *Tropical*, sold as 'exotic' or a *Blush* with the byline 'floral & flirty'. I gave Clare the choice: without a nanosecond's pause – flirty. But we never got round to flirting with the dry shampoo – she was just too tired. Maybe this was the spa-treatment-too-far. No 'Hostess' left in the poor old sis.

I realize that there is an essential simplicity needed for Clare now. Just talking to my Dear Lady Wife about this, and I came up with what I need to be. The three 'C's: Calm, Consistent and Capable. That is what I have to bring into her bedroom with me every time I enter. A gentle energy; making sure that everything is where it always has been, that there is a rhythm to the day no different to any other day; and that whatever new obstacle appears, it can be dealt with.

Too tired to attempt any physio today. Doesn't matter, as she nimbly moved from bed to wheelchair with ease. But we will try tomorrow.

Happy September and love to all.

Throwing shit outwards

2 SEPTEMBER 2016

My classmate at drama school, and flatmate for those three years, Ash, is now a vicar. Odd that I should be writing about Ash on this posting, as today, 2 September, is the birthday of the third member of our flat, Simon, who tragically drowned a couple of years after we left school. Happy birthday, Simon.

Ash, as a vicar, spends time with the dying, and a couple of weeks ago when he came to see me for the evening, gave me a useful piece of advice:

The dying person is the Centre. The First Circle around that, the close family. Next Circle, close friends. Then outwards, circle by circle to friends, people-you'd-be-happy-to-have-a-pint-with, people-you'd-send-a-Christmas-card-to, and outwards to the world at large…

And here's the advice: You are allowed to throw shit outwards, but not inwards. The person at the centre can throw as much shit as their energy allows – can toss it to the outer circles if they're able. Family can hurl excrement at friends, but none of us can throw shit inwards: friends not at close friends, close friends not at the family. And, above all, never at the Centre.

I liked that analogy. And I liked that a vicar used the word shit.

A few years ago I had lunch with a very interesting woman called Rose George who had just written a book called *The Big Necessity* about the enormous problem of sanitation in the Developing World. Almost all of the book looks at human excrement and how to deal with it effectively, so as not to contaminate the water supply and thus make the people sick. Over a rather nice lunch I asked her what word she would choose to use for our 'human waste' – and her answer, without pausing for thought, was 'shit'. So, shit it is. And apologies for offending anyone with the choice of word.

I raise this as I got a bit of shit thrown at me this morning from the Centre. We had just had a difficult time getting from the commode/wheelchair back into bed. Her legs buckled and I had had to try and lift Clare a little to get her onto the mattress, causing extreme discomfort and anxiety. I tried to apologize (not choosing the right moment, of course – just too soon after the trauma) and I got back, 'I'm in pain!' 'I understand,' I replied. 'NO, YOU DON'T!'

And, of course, I don't. I cannot in any way comprehend. I am not even in the neighbourhood, not even in the street, let alone with her in her House of Pain. And that is just the pain side of things – along with that comes the anxiety, fear, rage, frustration, helplessness...

We managed to calm down. She managed to rest. And then to discuss, briefly, what had happened between the two of us. I said I was trying as hard as I could. And she said that she was, too.

We are both trying. We are both human. We are in very, very different places of strength and health, but both occupying the same physical space, trying to navigate the situation with as much grace, love and humour as possible.

And sometimes it gets messy, but that is allowed, and we are allowed to get frustrated. We are allowed to get angry. But she is the only one of our pairing who is allowed to throw shit.

And that is as it should be.

Love to all.

Do you speak English?

3 SEPTEMBER 2016

For some odd reason I was sent two things today, and neither of them in English.

One, a four-line text on my phone in Latin – Googled, and found to be a poem by Hadrian – the other, a German magazine.

Both about death.

And it got me thinking: we don't speak Death in this country, do we? We don't learn it from our parents, we're not taught it at school. It is very rare to find people conversing in it, unless they are somehow 'specialists'.

When confronted by it, we mumble the couple of stock phrases we *have* learned – 'deepest sympathy' or 'condolences' – just like we would in a foreign country with a seemingly impenetrable language, where we will have learned 'please' and 'thank you'. (Or not, if you're me – one of the only things I can say in Polish is 'How much is the fridge?' and 'Because I'm Worth It' in Dutch . . .) Or do what just about every Brit does, when faced with a foreigner, say very slowly and very loudly, 'DO . . . YOU . . . SPEAK . . . ENGLISH ??'

We are mainly just embarrassed when encountering the language we don't understand, and grin idiotically, then get a bit angry that we are being made to feel embarrassed, then feel ashamed, as we are feeling angry at a person talking to us about death. I know, as I have done all these things: have felt so cross at having to write the 'condolences' letter, as I just don't know the words. The embarrassment comes, sometimes, when I tell folk what I'm doing at the moment – and they just *have* to tell me about something not *quite* as bad, but that has just happened to them, or a close friend of theirs... Embarrassment, pure and simple.

For a few years, I would go to a hospice in North London and do some comic Christmas readings. My dad's wonderful cousin Mervyn, who is as close to a saint as anyone I have ever known, was a regular hospice volunteer: playing the piano, organizing sing-alongs, quizzes, or just chatting to the folk there. He would drag me over every December for a good few years to entertain the outpatients after their Christmas lunch. I went willingly, but always terribly unsure as to how I should behave, how I should *be* in this place where the only reason people are there is because they are facing their death, not that far in the future.

I didn't really get over this issue until I started going to our local Marie Curie hospice with Clare in the last few months. But I will save my hospice musings for another blog.

Why can't we speak Death? Have we just forgotten it? I think we probably have – all wrapped up in our country's recent history of the rise of the 'Nuclear Family', of people leaving their childhood places and moving far away for work. Not that long ago, a household would comprise of Mum, Dad and children, plus, probably, a spinster aunt, a grannie or granddad. The old folk rubbing along with the toddlers – an interwoven, multi-generational family unit. And the aged would die at home, and every member of the family would have been a part of that death. Now, however, there are very few set-ups like this, and most of the older generation in the family end their time in 'homes' or in hospital. We don't witness the act of dying any more, let alone ever see a dead body.

Through both planning and fate, we are lucky enough to have a multi-generational family arrangement. My wife has moved about

200 metres since her birth; our house is opposite her mother's flat and Clare lives a dozen doors down the street. For many years we have had three generations sitting down to share a dinner every evening. My wife was brought up in a house (just a few doors up the street from where we live now) where her grannie lived with them for the seventeen years before she died: the subject of a wonderful book by Phyllida Law, Emma's mum, called *Notes to my Mother-in-Law*. Available anywhere, and a fantastic read. Along with her next one, *How Many Camels Are There in Holland?* – about her mum and dementia. Her third book will be available when she can be bothered to get round to finishing it...

Thus the language of death was alive and well in their family, as I hope it is in ours, now: that our daughter Gaia, if not fluent, is at least learning it. Which is a fantastically wonderful and healthy thing, as hard as it obviously is.

Clare is just quietly getting on with the days. She sleeps through them, mostly. Is still able to use the loo, take her meds, have a chat, see some chums, raise the odd smile and salute.

On present form, she will probably outlive me.

Love to all.

Nothing to do in the afternoon...

4 SEPTEMBER 2016

There's an old joke: Why doesn't an actor look out of the window in the morning? Because then he'll have nothing to do in the afternoon...

Funny.

Doesn't apply to me, though. I think I work harder when I'm 'resting' than I do when I'm on set. Maybe not 'work' – but I'm constantly engaged with a stream of tasks. I love to create, to be physical, to do stuff. I love to get to the end of a day and see something that wasn't on this planet at the start of the day – be it a piece of writing, a bit of woodwork, a painting, a planted-up vegetable garden, whatever.

This period of time I'm in doesn't allow for any of that. It is purely about being available – ready to spring into action when the bell goes, or gently wander into Clare's bedroom every hour or so to check that all is well. It is about waiting. In Clare's flat. And I'm finding this stasis really hard.

Clare is finding it hard, too. She needs to be *doing*. When gainfully employed, she would always be the first in the office and the last out, often working weekends as well. Both of us playing out what our parents instilled in us – the Work Ethic. I think our dad took it further, though: a phlegmatic Northern man, who rose from a working-class family to become a professor. His solution to any problem (even his advice to me, when heartbroken at eighteen), 'Get your head down' – knuckling down and working hard will solve everything...

We had a bit of a problem this morning at meds time – Clare was unable to swallow her pills. So, we did our usual: managed to get the tiny anti-anxiety pill down, had a snooze, and attempted again a while later. It was a success – but the usual routine of the day was out of kilter, and she was in the deep opiate sleep until about 4 p.m. When I managed to wake her, she was rather frustrated that most of the day had already passed. She needed more of a plan for the coming days.

She needed A LIST.

'I like to have a bit of a plan. It makes me feel like I'm involved with the world.'

I made the list: a wash, linen and outfit change, all pencilled in for tomorrow. Emails to be dictated. And there was one other thing, but it slipped her mind as she drifted off, mid-sentence.

Working hard. Being seen to work hard and achieve, in her mind, brought approval for Clare. And now that she cannot achieve, how does she get that approval? I think this is what's going on in the head of my sister now. When she has been told by all the health professionals that there will be no improvement, that where she is now is as good as it will ever be, she is still striving to achieve. Or maybe it's just more the Wise bloody-mindedness: 'I'll show them – I'll walk to the loo . . .'

And, of course, this search for approval-by-doing is just nonsense. We are loved for who we are, not what we do. I think Clare knows this now. But I think that it has taken this disease for her to really understand that. I *hope* she knows – the incredible amount of love that is all around her, both physically and in the ether via all of you is just too gargantuan to ignore.

Love to you all.

'To pee, or not to pee'

5 SEPTEMBER 2016

Sorry. Bad pun. But a serious point:

Clare is finding it increasingly difficult to have a pee. We had five failed outings to the loo yesterday, between lunch and bedtime.

Each attempt involves getting out of bed, standing, sitting on the uncomfortable plastic wheelchair/commode seat when there's not a lot of bum left to cushion, calming down, being wheeled into place over the loo, waiting, getting frustrated, admitting defeat, being wheeled back, standing, getting back into bed, calming down…

No fun at all.

Less fun, when the last unsuccessful outing was at 3 a.m. this morning.

Shebo, our nurse, thinks it's time for a catheter (a tube inserted into the bladder that drains the urine into a bag). A huge step for Clare. And something that I will have to 'seed' with her over the next days: raise the idea, let it sit with her, talk about it some more, wait… Just like I did with getting her the hospital bed. As these things – even though they help, lessen anxiety, make life easier or less painful – are all major 'Milestones on the Road' for her.

This posting is probably just an extension of yesterday's – Clare will not accept where she is and what is happening to her. She will constantly search for a solution, an alternative, a 'Second Opinion'. She continually questions everything. Which is great – it's what I've tried to instill in my daughter: don't accept the perceived wisdom, always question – but there comes a point where we just can't deny any more. Where we reach a 'watershed' on the journey. This is why it takes so long for me to persuade Clare to accept anything – whether it's the commode, the wheelchair, the hospital bed, or now the catheter – as these things are concrete; they're not ideas; they have physical form; and as such cannot be ignored or denied.

A reasonably busy day today. The meds went down without a fuss first thing this morning. Then the usual deep sleep. At lunchtime

Em came down the road and managed to give Clare a good wash – sitting in the commode/wheelchair in the bathroom, where she was sponged, soaped and dried, whilst I changed the bed-linen. Back to bed for a moisturize, a fresh set of pyjamas, and she was all ready for her afternoon Reiki session with our friend John.

Later on, now, and after another two failed attempts on the loo, I raised the idea of a catheter. No response. But it will be being processed somewhere in Clare's subconscious. We will, hopefully, have Shebo and Dr Phil here tomorrow to discuss it with her. I will have to make sure I keep 'seeding' the idea with her before they come. It may take a few days – it will take a lot of processing, that's for sure. And you can bet your bottom dollar that when Dr Phil talks about it, Clare will ask for a second opinion...

Love to all.

'Tough-icult'

6 SEPTEMBER 2016

Remember I wrote about compound nouns a few posts ago? Clare came up with her own this afternoon – it may have to become a family word from now on: 'Tough-icult' (and for those pedants out there, I know it's not a bloody noun...).

She was remarkable with Dr Phil and Shebo: focused, present, listening and responsive. But still unable to accept where she is. I did my usual, sitting quietly and making notes. What follows is as verbatim as possible...

Clare is aware that she's not getting any better, but has to find ways of helping herself: simple things – like getting up in the night and going to the loo by herself. A 'wee bit of autonomy' will make life less difficult. If she can move from A to B using sticks, she will feel self-controlled in terms of movement. She feels out of control: with what's going on and even what time it is. She needs a better clock. [*Already ordered via the Internet: date, month, day and time – in big digits and letters, to go on her over-bed table.*] And she looks to Dr Phil for advice.

Dr Phil navigated beautifully: the hardest thing is loss of control, and our task is to find where control and independence can be found. Within all this is the acceptance of a 'remorselessly progressive disease', and the acknowledgement that she has people to help – so, she should accept the help offered.

Clare is phenomenally frustrated. She feels claustrophobic as a result of being out of control. She panics about being dehydrated (even after being told that the meds she's on don't dehydrate; only cause her mouth to feel dry as they stop saliva being produced). She panics about the idea of making it to the loo by herself at night, and then getting stuck there.

Dr Phil suggested we look at energy and her 'waterworks': it becomes unmanageable, having fruitless trips to the loo. It is exhausting and frustrating. If she were to have a urinary catheter fitted, the 'upside' would be potentially more energy to spend on something else – like sitting on the sofa and chatting with friends.

Clare asked if we go the catheter route, are we *improving*?

It's taking a step back to maybe give us two steps forward, was the reply. And that she and I should mull it over...

I have tried to mull with Clare, but to no avail. Let's see how she feels about it in the morning. We have just had two unsuccessful trips to the loo. I have given her her evening meds, but she asks that I wake her before I go to bed, to have another attempt. I know that she is not worried about the 'medicalization' aspect of the catheter – that there will necessarily be nurses around more regularly. I think she is quite keen on the idea of a proper, professional 'bed-bath' – goodness knows, anything is better than her brother in his cheap knickers in the shower with her, or her sister-in-law wielding a sponge…

I tried to make light of it all by pointing out to Clare that I already have an age-old relationship with urine bags: when I was in my year off between school and university, I worked as a Community Service Volunteer – at Nottingham University, working primarily with a student with muscular dystrophy, but also responsible for helping a guy with paraplegia, and another with cerebral palsy. Urine bags were a daily ritual. That said, I understand the emotional enormity of the situation we are facing here.

However, someone who feels that they should be able to walk themselves to the loo, obviously doesn't need a catheter. It is purely the fact that we have not done enough physiotherapy that is stopping her perambulations. In 'practical terms', we need a 'daily physical'. A 9 a.m. workout, to allow her to 'tick things off the list that allow me to function *per se*'.

(Blimey. Even *she's* using Latin now – makes me feel like I should have paid more attention in Latin lessons at junior school, rather than just continually dropping my pencil so I could reach down, pick it up off the floor and try and see up the skirt of my Latin teacher…)

I am acutely aware that this is Clare's gig. To be run as she wants to run it. Whatever she feels will make things more bearable, less anxiety-provoking, I will try to facilitate. We have a new clock on the way; new straws ordered (as the ones we are using are a bit flimsy) and a new set of pyjamas. We will try a workout. And I will keep trying to 'seed' the idea of a catheter.

Sorry. This is all a bit brutal. For light relief, here are a couple of photos:

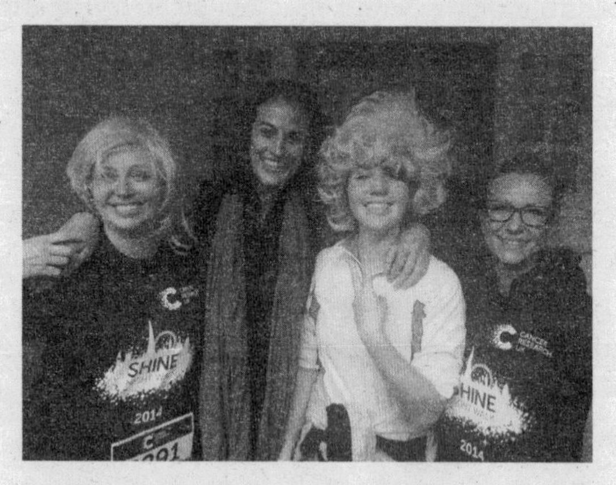

At our house, before the 'Shine' walk, 2014, for Cancer Research UK: Clare, Sandra, Gaia and Sarah

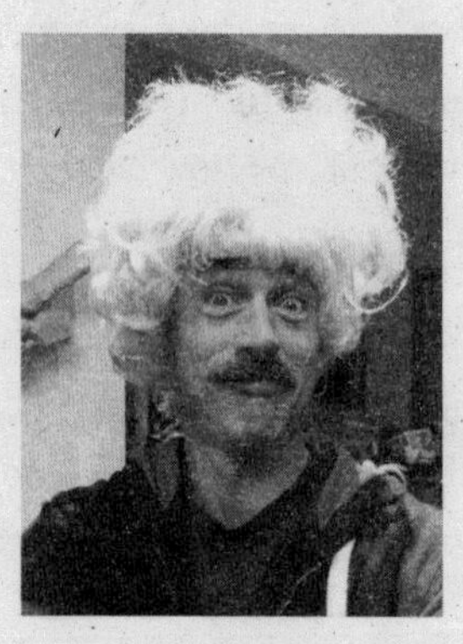

Me. In Gaia's wig. The facial hair was for a part. Honestly

Love to all.

'That's very nearly an armful!'

7 SEPTEMBER 2016

We had a wonderful British comedian from the mid-1950s to the early '60s, called Tony Hancock. He had a wildly popular radio show called *Hancock's Half Hour*. Both Clare and I are intimately aware of his work, as when we were children we had an LP (a long-playing record) of two of his shows: 'The Blood Donor' and 'The Radio Ham', which we played to death. In 'The Blood Donor', Hancock tries to do his civic duty and donate blood, but is appalled at the amount required:

Hancock: How much do you want then?

Doctor: Well, a pint, of course.

Hancock: A pint? Have you gone raving mad? I mean, I came here in all good faith, to help my country. I don't mind giving a reasonable amount, but a pint? Why, that's very nearly an armful!

This is a reasonably longhand way (and trying to be as discreet as possible) of raising the 'catheterization' of Clare this afternoon. Shebo and her colleague Gil came over, armed with various bits of kit, fortuitously coinciding with the latest failed attempt at peeing. After they had spent quite some time in the bedroom, only coming out to ask for new sheets, a towel, a plastic carrier bag and a tray, I was allowed in, and shown how to empty *the bag* – already containing 'more-than-an-armful'...

Bless her, Clare dealt with it all in the most stoic manner. It didn't make it any easier to be told that she was the easiest catheterization that Shebo had ever undertaken. It's horrid, whichever way you look at it: having a plastic tube coming out of you, filling a bag (hanging, at present in a ripped plastic carrier bag, tied to the bed base – I'll come up with a more elegant solution tomorrow). We got into a bit of a tangle this evening, though, when Clare thought she needed to go to the loo for the other reason – trying to work out how to attach the bag to the commode/wheelchair, and then getting tangled as she got back into bed…

All will become clear in time. We will get some tutoring in the fine art of tube-wrangling. We will also need a bit more help with washing – to minimize any risk of infection – and Clare is happy with the idea of district nurses coming round a few times a week to give her a bed-bath.

In a surreal mirror-image way, I'm experiencing what happened when our daughter was born. At first, all we needed were nappies. Then we needed a car-seat, a baby-carrier, a sling, a bath, bottles, a cot, a high chair… The extreme amount of kit needed for one tiny person was mind-boggling. And Clare and I are now facing a similar thing, but from a much darker angle: new pieces of kit turning up on a regular basis, as she is 'outgrowing' what we had before: the hospital bed replacing the inflatable pillow-raiser that was on her old bed; the commode/wheelchair replacing the wheeled Zimmer frame; a plastic tube replacing the need to physically go to the bathroom on the commode/wheelchair…

We have just finished the meds, put on bedsocks, I've filled her over-bed table with glasses of water, tonic, smoothie; made sure she has everything she needs, within reach. I wished her an unbroken night's sleep, and she started to wish me one in return, before realizing it was up to her whether I slept through the night or not.

We both need a good night's sleep. Let's hope the new plumbing paraphernalia allows it…

Love to all.

For whom the bell tolls

8 SEPTEMBER 2016

I am aware that the style of these postings is changing. Gone are the days of my whimsical thoughts. More now about procedures. More *medicalization*. Less personal. I will try and keep a bit of lightness about me in the upcoming words...

It was the World Premiere, last night, of *The Catheter*. I'd left enough liquids on the over-bed table to keep an entire lifeboat of shipwrecked sailors hydrated for a good month, so even Clare couldn't get through that many glasses. What could possibly go wrong?

The bell did not toll for me the entire night. So, what went wrong was that I had the worst night's sleep I've had since all this started: too hot, too cold, needed the loo, needed a drink, needed to check on Clare – exactly the same as the first night your baby sleeps through – you're certain the lack of crying means they're dead...

Clare *did* get through that many glasses, but thankfully the catheter did its job perfectly, and a football-shaped bag greeted me first thing. We managed to wrangle the tubing, make her comfortable, and she spent the morning in her usual deep sleep.

Our lovely GP, Miranda, came over for a visit mid-afternoon, as she hasn't clapped eyes on Clare for months. Clare did her usual 'Hello! How *are* you?' I left them to it for a good quarter of an hour. Miranda rejoined me in the living room, astounded with the conversation they'd just had, but trying to balance it with the obviously huge physical deterioration since she'd last seen Clare.

I was wrong to think a chat with a GP might exhaust the sister – she wanted to lie on the sofa (as we'd made that a plan-for-the-day this morning) and spend some time with Rose, who'd come over to chum her. Fortunately the day was lovely, so Clare was able to look out at the sunny garden, still in flower in parts, whilst getting Rose to make a list of phone calls she wanted to make over the next days.

I was thrilled this afternoon to receive a call telling me that we had been fast-tracked into an NHS Complete Care Package: both nursing care for Clare and respite care for me. Potentially twenty-four-hour. Wow. Louise, the lady calling, was adamant that I have daily care set up as soon as possible – both as she knew I was trying to shoulder the load on my own, and also as it's important to set up a quotidian (is that Latin?? See – I *was* paying attention) rhythm with Clare; just so she doesn't really notice when the daily care becomes essential rather than just welcomed. Louise is coming over on Tuesday – she normally arranges everything on the phone, but I stressed to her that Clare needs to be a part of any arrangements.

We had a Good Day. Clare's clock turned up and is hanging prominently on the wall by the bed: so she knows time, day, date, month. She's sporting a new, roomy cotton pyjama top. She has had a good deal of time present and focused. She's had a list made. And I have been thrown a potential lifeline in the form of a Complete Care Package. A part of me wanted to shrug off any help offered, but I know that I am only a mammal. Not a superhero. I've no cape. I'm a brother trying to do the best for his sister. And really, at the end of the day, what do I know about palliative care? Not a great deal, although I'm learning fast. And there is, undoubtedly, a great deal of collateral damage to all this, which I have to be needful of.

To know when to act, is the thing. I remember hearing a very interesting radio programme, some time back, about the Iraq invasion, I think. Stuffed with pundits and army folk. And one guy really stood out for me – his opinion was that, actually, the easiest course of action is to rush in, all guns blazing. And it takes more guts to do nothing (if 'nothing' is the best course of action, which it sometimes is). I have always been the 'all guns blazing' kind of guy, the make-it-up-as-you-go-along bloke. Which has served me reasonably well over the years, but with a bit of age (all right, a *lot* of age) you get to know your limitations, the moments where pause is needed. I feel now that I am close to my limit. I am not ashamed of that. I *need* professional help. Clare needs professional help.

Oh, dear. I haven't done very well on the whimsy, have I?? To make amends, a couple of photos. A trip we all made to South Africa, back in 2007. Bit of a safari and a bit of a talk at the Market Theatre in Johannesburg. Can't remember what the talk was about – film-making, perhaps? Suffice to say, a couple of gorgeous photos of the gorgeous sister in full flow…

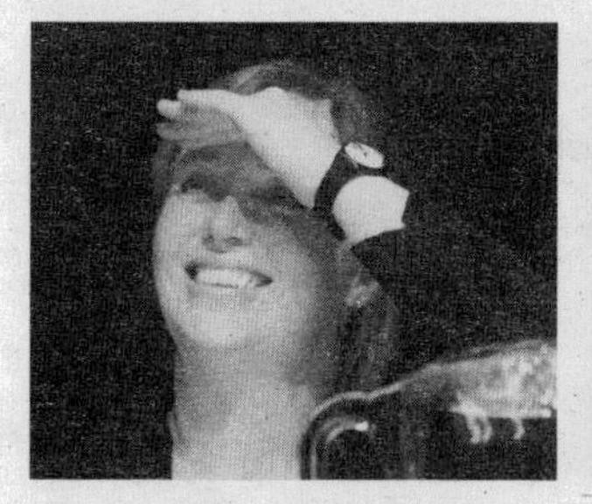

Taking a question from the audience

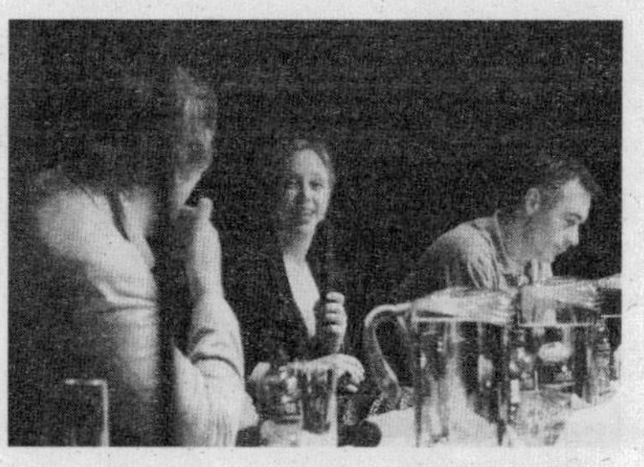

Answering the question. A Rose between the Two Thorns Stephen Fry and me…

Love to all.

'Why, where are you going?'

9 SEPTEMBER 2016

After the wonderful premiere of *The Catheter*, I'm afraid to say it did not live up to its reviews... Somehow, mid-morning, the tube and its attachment parted company.

After a hasty pyjama change, an unplanned trip on the commode/ wheelchair to the loo, frantic bed-stripping, washing, disinfecting, drying, fresh linens and re-settling, I realized that all this is very much now 'above my pay-grade'. A call to Louise of the NHS carers: district nurse to visit as soon as possible to check the catheter (I'd managed to plug the air-gap, but was not utterly confident, although had decided against the gaffer tape solution for now), and a hasty arranging of two carers' visits per day over the weekend – first thing in the morning for an hour for a wash, and last thing in the evening just to check everything's fine.

Once the lovely district nurse had been and made sure the catheter was working, I told Clare of the weekend's care plan – and got back, 'Why? Where are *you* going?'

Hmmmmm. As gently as I could I pointed out that she had asked for professional washing and 'intimate care' and that I also needed some respite.

It may be a tricky meeting on Tuesday with Louise, Clare and me. I understand completely that when faced with the chronic, painful and terminal illness that Clare is enduring, there is little energy available, or even interest, in looking outwards. That the day is necessarily self-absorbed. And I have been the constant over the last months: available, day or night, at the ring of a bell. Which, I must stress, I have wanted, just as much as Clare.

The uncharted territory that we have been navigating over the last number of weeks, trying to keep a steady course, facing square-on the new obstacles together, and in the main, solving the steady stream of new issues, has now come to a head. Medicalization is starting to overtake the purely dispensing-of-meds/physical needs that, thus far, I have been able to serve.

Some years ago, a wonderful American friend of mine, James, was working with an outfit called the Heffter Institute, studying the help that LSD can give to the terminally ill – specifically in the alleviation of fear and anxiety. I'm just gently wondering, now that it's all getting a bit *real* for Clare, whether I shouldn't just go down to Soho and try and score some serious hallucinogenics for her. Just a thought. If the reality of the situation is untenable, thus being denied, why not create an *alternative reality*?

Like the Woody Allen quote (or, something like it, anyway), 'I don't mind the idea of death, I just don't want to be there when it happens.'

He may have a point.

Love to all.

—

Compassion Fatigue

10 SEPTEMBER 2016

Compassion Fatigue

> Noun: *'Indifference to charitable appeals on behalf of suffering people, experienced as a result of the frequency or number of such appeals.'*

That's what I always thought it was. But did you know that there's a Compassion Fatigue Awareness Project – and nothing to do with the above indifference?

This is what they say on their website:

> *'Caring too much can hurt. When caregivers focus on others without practicing self-care, destructive behaviors can surface. Apathy, isolation, bottled up emotions and substance abuse head a long list of symptoms associated with the secondary traumatic stress disorder now labeled: Compassion Fatigue.'*

Well, I've happily ticked off all of their destructive behaviours. Especially the substance abuse. But then I was an abuser before I started being a full-time carer, so maybe I'm just a drunk and should ignore that as a pointer...

That said, it's comforting to know that I am exhibiting signs of an accepted *secondary traumatic stress disorder* – and not just being a grumpy old arse.

I suppose it's not rocket science to realize that the carer can start to mirror the person they're caring for. Purely the amount of time spent in a situation must create a transference between the two parties involved. If Clare feels isolated, not in control, feeling the loss of identity that an active participation in the wider world had given her, marginalized, it's no wonder I'm feeling these things as well (of course, in a hugely less existential way), after ten weeks of 24/7...

So what can we do?

I've done a great deal of reading over the last months about terminal illness and mortality, and just now, stumbled across a paper called 'Hope in the Terminally Ill'.

I think it's interesting to share with you all a few choice words from it:

> *'Mortality is suddenly confronted, and the concept of hope wanes as the unattainable goal of extended life vanishes... But a seemingly paradoxical question arises: because hope is frequently defined as the expectancy of good in the future, how can a future defined in hours, days, weeks, and months provide hope?*
>
> *'When first confronted with a terminal illness, most patients typically relate hope to a tangible treatment or cure that can prolong existence despite overwhelming information to the contrary.*
>
> *'The obstacles that hinder hope: abandonment and isolation, uncontrolled pain, and devaluation of personhood.*
>
> *'Sources of hope: including family, friends, health care professionals, and God or a higher spiritual being.*
>
> *'In the context of a terminal illness, hope can exist even when time is limited. Such hope is bolstered by appreciating the patient's value, strengthening and reconciling their relationships with family and friends.*
>
> *'Although physicians may find it hard to comprehend, when everything seems to be lost, that hope may actually be stronger than ever before.'*

I feel that this is the key to our present situation. Clare went all-guns-blazing (it's obviously a family trait) at treating this disease. She tried everything – all the chemotherapy and radiation; surgery; a month at an Indian Ayurvedic clinic; seeing a healer; being on a clinical trial. Even when she was so ill, a few weeks ago, she was still contemplating aggressive intravenous chemotherapy. All hope-based.

Being told that the time for treatment was over brought with it the loss of hope. This is clear. And try as I may, I am unable to focus her outwards in any way – no possibility of what was written about in the paper of *strengthening and reconciling relationships with family and friends.* And I cannot help with this. This is something that may or may not materialize. It will not happen, I believe, until she comes to terms with where she is.

I was wrong, I think, in yesterday's post to say that Clare's locked-in state is purely to do with her physical illness. I think now it is much more to do with the *loss of hope.*

And hope is so powerful. We had a Woody Allen quote yesterday, today another great comic depressive, John Cleese, from his film *Clockwise*: 'It's not the despair. I can take the despair. It's the hope I can't stand.'

Amen to that.

We had our first visit this morning – bright and early, 7.45 a.m. – from Kyle and Laura from Carelink. Before Laura had even got through the front door of the building, she let loose, 'I'm such a *huge* fan!!' I suppose I'd forgotten that I'd ever had an existence outside this flat... You see?? *Loss of identity*...

They gave Clare a proper bed-bath and then started to go through all the paperwork required to set up her Care Plan. Unsurprisingly, mid box-ticking, she fell asleep, so we did the admin without her. All very thorough. And knowing that we have professionals on call – twenty-four hours a day if we need them – is very comforting for me.

It's not nice to feel grumpy with your dying sister, and I'm glad I've been able to discover that I'm not just a bad person, but that my grumpiness has a name: Compassion Fatigue. And maybe now there is some hope for both of us in the potential support on offer.

Although Clare had me cancel this evening's visit of the carers...

Love to all.

Reality Mortality

11 SEPTEMBER 2016

There was a game show on the TV in the 1970s when I was a kid called *The Krypton Factor* – referencing (I assume) Superman's home planet of Krypton and thus suggesting that the contestants needed superpowers to undertake the challenges set – mental agility, physical ability, high intelligence.

I'm thinking of getting in touch with Endemol (the crowd who make *Big Brother*) to see if I can sell them an immersive television reality show. Called – I don't know – *Terminal!* or maybe *Big Sister* (a tad too specific perhaps??). *Reality Mortality* – I like that one. OK, *Reality Mortality* it is.

On *Reality Mortality* we will have a group of disparate folk – all living in a house together, all being tasked to care for a terminally ill patient. Nobody can leave the house. Everyone has to do their share of washing up. New daily challenges – stretching their physical and mental ability and intelligence. A 'Diary Room' where they can bang on about the stresses of compassion fatigue, and their personal difficulties with their fellow carers. (Maybe they are all dressed in a kind of army combat outfit – called, for the purposes of our format, compassion fatigues. Or is that a gag too far??) One by one they will be voted off by the viewers, for things like forgetting to empty the bag, not being able to work out how the two physical therapy 'slider sheets' work in tandem (I had to show our nurses how to make the hospital bed – they had never seen such sheets . . .), not being able to come up with ideas of how to open the individually wrapped Effentora pills (see post from 31 August).

It'll be HUGE. I'm already working on my acceptance speech at the BAFTAs.

No, no, but seriously, folks . . . what Clare and I are going through is an hour-to-hour *Krypton Factor* challenge. We had the morning visit from the Carelink pair. I set them the challenge of washing Clare's hair in bed (for someone who can't turn their head in any direction). A challenge too far, it seems. Clare was stressed, the carers were not allowed to put her onto the commode to wheel her to the bathroom, as that is not in her 'care plan', so I sent them away, and have cancelled any care until we have the Big Meet on Tuesday. I gave the sis an anti-anxiety pill, and went onto the Internet:

How . . . to . . . wash . . . hair . . . without . . . water . . .

Various things appeared: baby powder, rubbing alcohol, lemon juice, vinegar, spray shampoos. Then I discovered no-rinse shampoo: just rub in, watch it lather, and towel it out. Wow. But it gets better. From a health-care site: the 'no-rinse shampoo cap' – looks like a shower cap, but contains the shampoo inside. Just take it out of the packet, put the cap on the head, massage it, take it off and towel dry. I have ordered three.

Managed to get out for a few minutes to do some shopping. Went to big local DIY superstore and got rather confused at the various receptacles available. Didn't quite have the courage to ask the passing Polish store worker which one they thought would be optimal for collecting urine when I empty Clare's bag.

I chose a washing-up bowl.

The lovely Fiona and her hubby, Richard, came over to throw me out this afternoon. Bliss. Until I got to cocktail hour at my house – opened up the fridge to get a beer, and was confronted with concrete proof that I have been away from home for too long: my beer drawer was full of salad. (I must ask Shebo what that is in Swahili, and add it to my collection of useful foreign phrases.)

We had a gorgeous, if brief, moment together as a family again. Gaia cooked steak, had made a wondrous collection of side dishes, and we shared a family meal. A quick trip down the road to give Clare her meds, and back up for a few games of backgammon with Gaia, then a moment in my study. Which is in absolute chaos.

I did, however, find an old newspaper article. 'Relative Values' from one of the Sunday magazines that Clare and I had done, probably in the late 1990s. A couple of lovely photos:

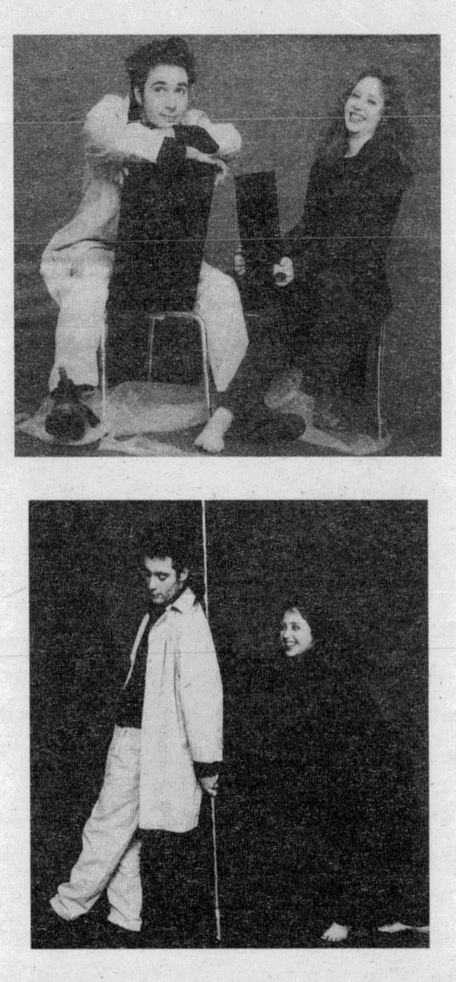

And a selection of what we said in the article, starting with Clare:

> *'Greg is absolutely my best friend. I was eighteen months old when he was born, and apart from university we have hardly ever been apart. He found my flat for me, he built my kitchen, and until nine months ago, he lived with me. My mum can count on one hand the times we've argued, and in fact I can remember each of those times... I feel safer with*

Greg than with anyone else. If we were in medieval times he'd be a good person to be with – he'd fight off the dragons and evil spirits. He likes to protect and he likes to love... and when I'm with him I feel special and loved too.'

And what I said:

'She is possibly the most caring person I know. She's got such a good heart that can easily be abused... she has to take everything on her shoulders and make sure everyone is all right. I think a lot of the time she is looking for approval. She has to realize that she isn't responsible for everybody else's happiness... To be honest, I can't see anyone not liking her, because she'll try so hard to overcome any problem... Boyfriends and girlfriends come and go, but we're brother and sister for life, and you can't mess that around.'

So, there we are. A reaffirmation of everything. A serendipitous moment, to have come across this article. True then, true now.

Love to all.

The roadie muses

12 SEPTEMBER 2016

After whatever latest moment of crisis has been overcome, our days meld seamlessly, one into the next. The rhythms of medicating, hydrating, emptying the bag, trying a bit of a conversation before the eyes roll back into the head, going to the shops for provisions, making up smoothies and watermelon juice, medicating, hydrating, emptying the bag...

I tried to mess with today's rhythm by beavering away with phone calls and emails. I finally confronted Clare this morning with what she actually wants from her days. What those in the know call her *goals*. Whether she wanted to see mates other than the A-Team Girls (Philippa Perry and Rose Smith who joined Clare at my school in the sixth form back in the early 1980s; Emma Clarke who was a fellow film-industry mate for over twenty years and Fiona Thomas who arrived via various Australian connections in the last century) who pop in and out at will. It is her old friend Jules's birthday today and I asked her if she were able at least to talk to her on the phone. So we did a test: putting the landline phone on speaker and calling my mobile. Seemed to work, and I called Jules, so they could have a chat. It went to voicemail. Ah, well. We tried.

It is a question of a trade-off between sedation and pain. The drugs ease the pain, but being a blunt instrument, they heavily sedate. Alongside this is the 'burden' of her illness bringing prolonged sleeping. So, my task today on our *Krypton Factor* was to try and find out whether there is a way of guaranteeing a moment of wakefulness in the day that can be shared. Clare is most available, clear and present between 3.00 and 5.00. In the morning. Not great, unless she wants to speak with her Australian chums. So is there a way of flipping this to 3–5 p.m.??

Emails banged off to various doctors. Phone calls to the palliative nurse. And I await any form of guidance. Maybe I will simply be told what Clare has been repeatedly told by Dr Phil on his visits here: that there will only be 'windows' which have to be seized. And we will never be able to plan when they will come.

I also attempted to raise what we want to talk about with Louise tomorrow. How we imagine we will use the care on offer. But Clare wasn't willing to engage. I will try again. And it's not just that she is finding it hard to sanction anyone other than her brother being here – she said to Rose, this afternoon, that she is aware that I need time away. She hasn't said that to me, though. Maybe she just can't start that conversation, as she's scared where it might go. So I have to start making unilateral decisions, which seems unfair, as she is desperate for a sense of control – at the same time unwilling to participate in the conversation. A dichotomy that I am unable to solve.

I'm being hard on her. I cannot even begin to imagine what she is trying to process in her head. And, once again, I know I am bringing my sheet music to someone else's recital, and have to keep repeating to myself: IT'S HER GIG. I am merely her roadie.

Sorry. This isn't as much fun as yesterday's post.

Love to all.

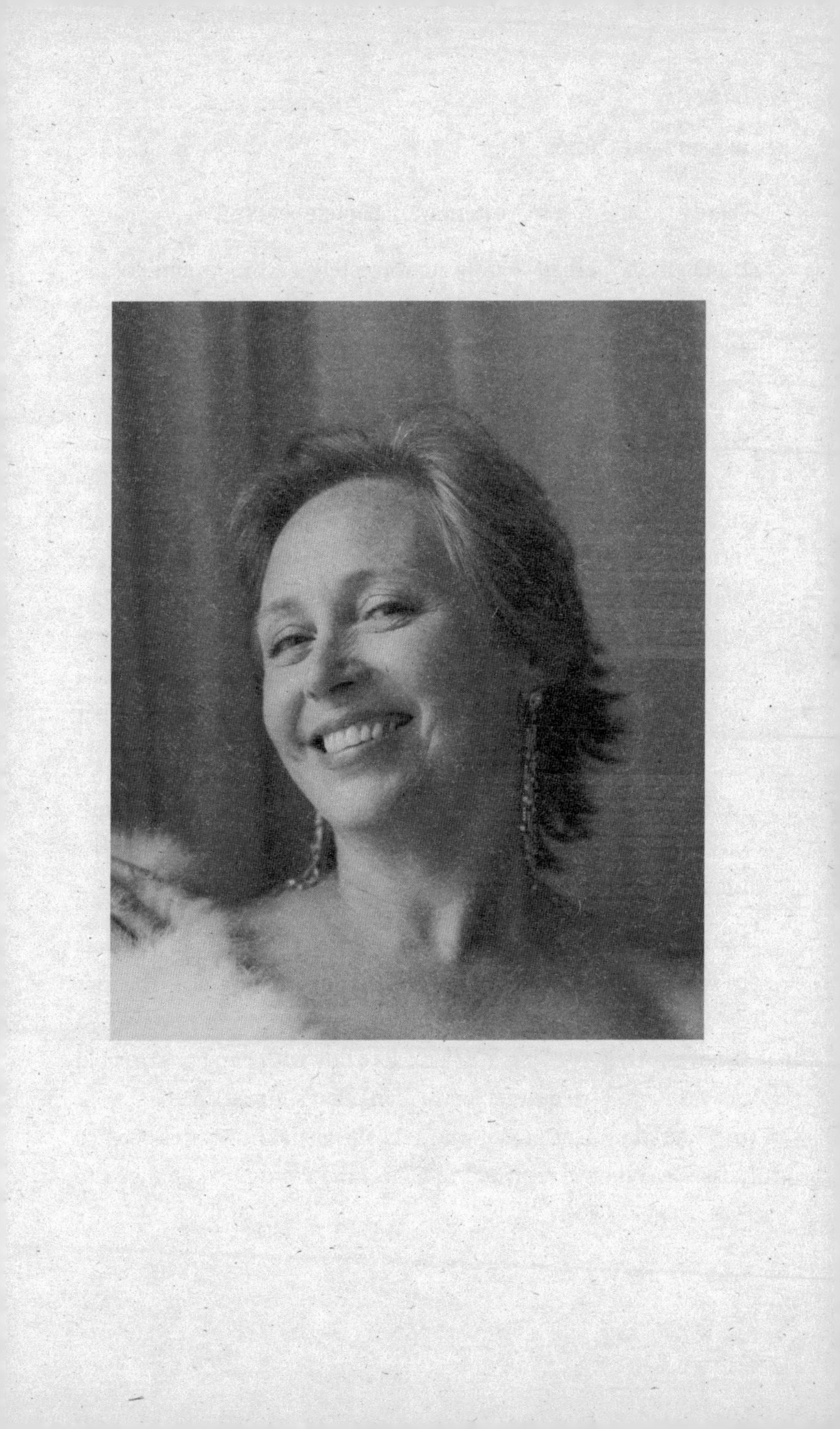

Clare

14 SEPTEMBER 2016

Clare died at 8.10 a.m. yesterday, 13 September 2016.

Ironically, or perhaps totally appropriately, within minutes of me posting the previous evening's blog about the 'sameness of days' and that I was going to have to make a unilateral decision, Clare was busy making other plans.

She was not her usual self in the early evening – the rhythm of the days had always been that by 7 or 8 p.m. she would have her smoothie, take the collection of meds, and then gently slide off into a big sleep. But that evening was different: she couldn't get comfortable, kept ringing the bell and getting me to rearrange her pillows, change the angle of the bed-base, try and move her on the mattress. We had exhausted the possibility of more opiates, so I gave her an Effentora – usually guaranteed to knock her out – but she was still bell-ringing for some time after.

At 10.30 I checked on her. She was asleep. I gave Grably his fifteenth meal of the day, he took himself to the door and I let him out for the night. I put myself to bed, hoping for as calm a night as possible.

I woke at 1 a.m. hearing noises and went to Clare's room. She was in some distress. Wide-eyed with hugely dilated pupils. Shallow, quick panting, every breath bringing with it a forcefully vocalized 'I can't... I can't... I can't...' I tried to talk with her, but she could not respond. I tried to get her to drink, but she was unable. I went to phone the night nurse, who said she would be over as soon as possible. When I returned to Clare, the words had changed to 'OK... OK... OK...'

Only with hindsight I realize that this was perhaps the frantic interior dialogue playing itself out.

Fifteen or so minutes later, Heather and Emma, the night nurses, arrived. I had a collection of meds that had been ordered some weeks ago (when we had thought to give Clare a big sedative for her nights, but had decided against it). Heather concocted the sedative and painkillers on offer, and gave Clare an injection. Within a few minutes she was calm and her eyes closed. I left her at about 3 a.m., calmly sleeping.

By 7 a.m. or so, she was back to being wide-eyed. But now totally unresponsive and immobile. Just an indistinct vocalizing on every breath.

We have an extraordinary backup. The fridge door is covered with telephone numbers for nurses, palliative care, 'Twilight Nursing' (until 11 p.m.) and the night nurses until 7 a.m. But, and I have no idea how this could not have been spotted, between about 7 a.m. and 9 a.m., there is nobody available. I called a number and was told to phone our NHS generic helpline: 111. There you get an operator, who is not medically trained. She said she had to go through a list of questions with me – was Clare bleeding?? After a pointless number of minutes of mindless questioning I was put on hold and then told I was being transferred to a nurse. Finally we managed to speak, but all she could suggest was that I call Camden GP cover. They may be there at 8 a.m. (not a lot of use to me at 7.30). On a whim I phoned Heather, the night nurse – she was no longer working, but would arrange a 'Rapid Response' nurse to come.

8 a.m. now. Back at the bedside.

I wiped Clare's face. I held her hand. I kissed her forehead. I told her I loved her. I said how unbelievable we had both been, but I said it was all just getting too fucked-up now. I told her that she didn't have to worry, that everything was sorted. And I told her that she could go now, if she wanted to.

I kept her hand in mine, and she died about a minute later.

Of course, once again, I had not understood. Once again, I had thought that this was my gig, that I was the one who would make the unilateral decision. Which was nonsense.

The unilateral decision was always Clare's to make. And she made it. Tuesday 13th was the day that would mark the change. The day of organizing the care package. The day that medicalization, procedures, professionals and strangers would start to creep in and take over our quiet space. Clare, obviously, could not countenance that. And I would like to believe that her leaving at this point was also an act of love for me, as she knew that I really couldn't countenance this unfolding new chapter either.

So she wielded the only power left to her. The power to excuse herself from the set-up. And what extraordinary power that was to behold. The power of her mind.

Clare has always been driven by her mind. She never really had a relationship with her body, with her physicality. So it is no surprise that what was happening to her body, what terrible wasting and swelling and pain – even though that was physically so debilitating – was not what took her away. *She* took herself away. Her 'self', her mind, brain, intellect, whatever you want to call it. That's what had kept her going for so long in this terrible disease, and that is what called the halt. With such Grace, Power and Spirit.

All she needed was to know that I fully sanctioned her wish. And the extraordinary nature of her brain – that in this situation, seemingly totally unresponsive, she heard me, and acted with such swift decisiveness.

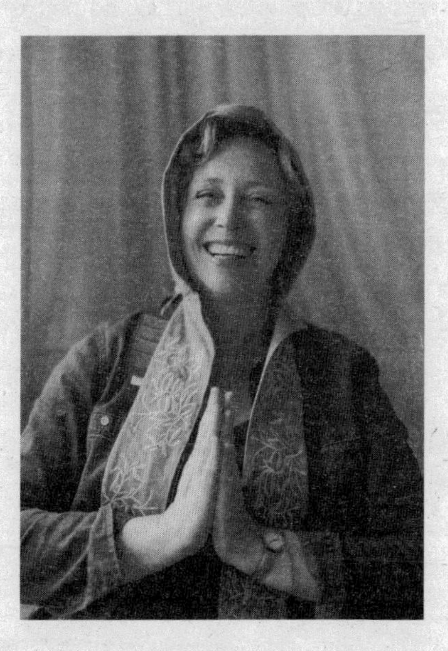

And, of course, as Death and Comedy are natural bedfellows, there were necessarily a few darkly humorous moments afterwards:

To start with I had to make sure Clare *was* dead: that there was no pulse. I held her wrist: nothing. Just to be sure, I held *my* wrist: nothing. Exactly what had happened a few years ago when Clare and I were with our mum when she died, I was unable to find a pulse on any of us... and I allowed myself a laugh with Clare now, as we both had a good laugh back then.

Within minutes of Clare's death, the phone went. It was the Rapid Response nurse. I told her Clare had just died: 'Oh – and I'm *already in the car*!' I quickly assessed whether being British meant that I had to apologize for my sister's death to someone I didn't know as we had upset their travel plans, but decided I didn't have to.

And when Em was on the phone to our local funeral directors, she said who she was and was greeted by, 'Is it your *mum*?'

None of the above, however, gets close to the craziness when I went to register my mum's death in York. It was the day after her death, and I had driven into town and parked in a big car park. As I got out, I bumped into her GP, who had signed her death certificate the day before. We talked for a number of minutes, and as she left and I turned to go to the registry office, I was accosted by a man holding a microphone:

'Greg? It's Greg Wise, isn't it? You're live on BBC Radio York.' (The car park is overlooked by the radio station.) 'What are *you* doing here?'

'I'm registering my mother's death.'

Without even the slightest pause: 'What's in the pipeline? Anything coming up? How's Emma?'

Again, I had to quickly check my being-British-appropriate response. Do I thump him? Ignore him and walk off, or answer his question?

I spent the next few minutes 'live on Radio York'...

I hope Clare would be proud of me. Some weeks ago I gathered the A-Team together and we went through her contacts, emails, my contacts and whoever the Girls could think of, and put together a 'phone cascade' – apportioned between us. I was desperate that we do this properly, that nobody who ought to receive a personal communication about Clare's death should find out via social media, or any other public platform. I was, for a nanosecond, 'Clipboard Greg'. Within an hour of Clare dying, the cascade started, and the reason that I didn't post anything yesterday was that not everybody who needed to be told *had* been told. Esther in Antarctica was still unaware... I managed to have a long chat with her this morning, but she already knew via the Aussie contingent. And apologies to whoever wrote in the 'comments' bit on the previous post, leaving their commiserations – I deleted them. Trying to manage the appropriate-information flow in this age is really hard. And, whoever reads this and feels upset that they had not been personally informed ahead of this public note – I sincerely apologize. We all tried our best.

So what now? Clare left her flat around lunchtime yesterday with a couple of kind (and terribly well-dressed) gents from the funeral directors. I registered her death at our council registry office in town (where the computer system was down, so was unable to get a certificate) and have arranged for Grably the cat to go to his new home. He was, of course, discombobulated by the day. We sat him on Clare after she had died, but he wasn't interested – no Greyfriars Bobby he – instead went to sleep on his chair. But once Clare had been taken away, he left the flat, and has been in the garden ever since – just coming in for food, and then leaving. Luckily it is beautiful weather, still – 91 degrees yesterday (33 Celsius) and balmy nights. This evening the lovely Emma Clarke (one of the A-Team) is coming to pick him up. She had Grably's brother and sister for many years, now both dead, but still has four cats, down in the countryside, so hopefully our furry friend will be happy in his new home. I've got together all his 'kit' – travelling basket, scratching post, bowls, litter tray – to go with him so he can feel some sense of continuity. Bless him – even I (by no means a cat-lover) have become very fond of this old gentleman. May he live out his remaining years in the same state of pampered bliss that his first eighteen have afforded him.

As Clare didn't talk to any of us about funeral plans or anything, we are having to work out what is most appropriate for this most unconventional girl. The feeling is that we won't have a funeral. Instead we will have a party. On her birthday – 19 November. A Saturday, fortunately. Start with an 'open mike' so whoever can say whatever they want. And then major dancing and drinking. For those of you who didn't know (can there be anyone?) Clare was a HUGE fan of 1980s Disco. So that's what we'll have. Start sorting out your outfits.

I'll post everything when we've decided. Along with donations to charities, for those of you who would like to do that.

This is a long post. Which is fitting, as you have all been on our journey, and needed to know the ending.

I will keep writing, as I have found this to be so helpful on so many levels. The enforced stasis that this has brought, although so hard for me, has also allowed me to sit and think and try to articulate the myriad thoughts bouncing around. And even though this has been, on paper, about the journey to Death, I think it is more about the journey of Life. About living, about people, about relationships, about the *essence* of all things. And, I think, has reinforced a few things that maybe all the noise and endless movement of my life has made me forget:

Live as honestly with yourself as possible; live to allow the moments not to go by unnoticed and uncelebrated; try to be kind both to yourself and those around you; try to find a way to love and be loved; keep asking questions, keep trying to find answers; but know when to stop.

And with that, I will stop. For now. But leave you with this. Pretty much sums things up:

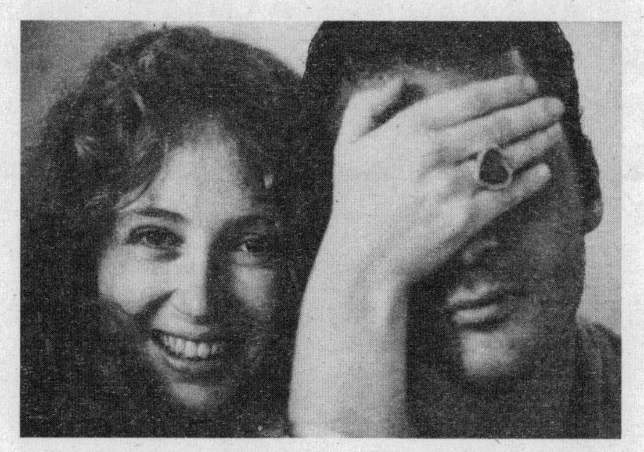

Love to all.

Emma and Gaia

18 SEPTEMBER 2016

Nothing of what you have all been reading over the last months – the total immersive care for my sister – would have been possible without the utter, unquestioning love and support of the two most incredible people in my life: my wife and daughter, Emma and Gaia.

No, that isn't right. Not *support* – their *equal* shouldering of the burden alongside me.

Witnessing a father and husband absenting himself, by choice, from the family for so long, with total understanding and grace.

I can write about this aspect of things, now that the daily care of my sister has come to an end. It did not seem right before this moment: muddying the waters in some way, opening up to view the primary dynamic in my life, running as a parallel story to this one, and necessarily on hold.

This 'holding pattern' started last summer. Literally a couple of days before we were all meant to go off on a wonderful holiday to Greece – Emma, Gaia, Clare and I.

Emma had organized a two-week cruise, just the four of us on a yacht, round some of the Greek islands – two days before we were all meant to go, Clare got the diagnosis of bone cancer. And that the treatment had to start right away.

I explained to Gaia that Clare just needed an operation on her broken arm (which was true, but only part of the story) so she wouldn't worry, but to cut a long story short, Clare and I didn't cruise round the Greek islands last summer...

Clare was originally diagnosed with breast cancer in 2013, her treatment continuing until the early months of 2014. We managed a wonderful fiftieth birthday celebration for her that November. (Ironically, the one who had organized it all was unable to be there – Emma was in New York, as her close friend Mike had just died.) Within a few months, however, Clare was in pain again. Those of you who have followed this blog from its inception will know the story, but suffice to say that for many months she carried around a number of pathological fractures – all mistreated by the various professionals she visited, until the summer of 2015.

Since then it has been an almost constant stream of hospitals, clinics and procedures – the family focused totally on Clare. And when I couldn't be with her for whatever appointment, Emma was at her side.

By the start of this year, Clare was on oral chemotherapy, and thus not tied to regular hospital visits. To make the most of this state of affairs, in February, Emma took her to an Ayurvedic clinic in India: she stayed a fortnight, and Clare a month. A shame, in hindsight, that she didn't write more fully about her stay there as it was such a powerful time: the day she got back to London I told her that I had *never* seen her looking so wonderful – beautiful, healthy, full of life. But she went to bed the next day, and never really got out of it again.

It was on this trip to India, just the two of them munching dhal and getting treatments, that wonderful conversations happened: nobody else to get in the way and time to explore thoughts fully. Perhaps the most potent was Clare's admission that she wished she 'had let love into her life'. She had an extraordinary amount of love in her life – she knew that – but not *that* kind of love…

Clare protected herself from the hurt that she knew naturally came hand in hand with *that* kind of love. She allowed herself to love and be loved, but probably, and essentially for her, *on her terms*: the love of friends, her family, colleagues, Grably and me.

And our relationship, as I am sure you are all aware if you've been following this blog, is not your archetypical brother/sister one. Clare and I were brought to an incredible closeness by the reasonably tricky family dynamic we grew up in, but we went opposite ways as a result: me looking for *that* kind of love – Clare shunning that and going the route of self-sufficiency: with her brother on hand, of course, to do whatever 'man things' needed doing. Probably the perfect set-up for her – someone to do the DIY without demanding a kiss afterwards…

She did, though, make demands of me – which I was always happy to honour; but having a family of my own meant their sanctioning of this arrangement – which was always given. Emma, and latterly Gaia, being so gracious, wise and understanding about the complex relationship that was *Me and Clare*.

Never more apparent than the moments after Clare's death. Emma and Gaia at the bedside within minutes, and the start of our family grieving. Oddly, or perhaps fittingly, the first real moment back as our family unit was the sharing of grief. An incredibly potent and positive thing for the three of us, and something that we will continue, as a family.

Emma lit scented candles and set them in the bedroom; Gaia cut flowers from the garden and put them in a vase on Clare's over-bed table, and while we waited for Dr Miranda to come and do her paperwork, she went out and returned with pastries and coffee. She went into a food-creating frenzy for the rest of the day. Obviously well brought up, or well versed with what to do in a time of death – we are all emotional, exhausted, our blood sugar dives – we need feeding.

Over the next couple of hours she put together the most fantastic buffet at home, which we decimated over the remainder of the day. Practicality – that's what is so important at these times and a true Act of Love.

And now we have to re-engage. Have to get back together as a family again. Start to repair the inevitable 'collateral damage'. It will take time, as it has been a long time in the making. And I feel that the grieving process will be a large part of the healing.

Interesting thing, grief. As I mentioned in an earlier blog, my close friend and flatmate over the three years at drama school, Simon, drowned when he was twenty-five. I was in a play at the time at the Nottingham Playhouse – far away from any of our school-mates, far away from the city we had all shared. Very much adrift. I went to see a sort of mystic lady in Nottingham, who told me that if I didn't grieve I would get physical heart problems. But try as I could, grief would not come. I gave up acting, I took myself to Australia, a friend joined me a few months later and the two of us rented a car and did a 10,000-kilometre journey in four weeks (and of course she couldn't drive . . .). Halfway through – on an endlessly straight road in the middle of the most enormous, flat, arid landscape I had ever found myself in – I started to cry . . . Maybe I just needed a sense of perspective. A sense of where I fit into the 'grand scheme of things'. I don't know. But I grieved. Big time.

Grief comes easier for me now, and I have found myself over the last few days, walking through Clare's flat, carrying boxes, suddenly overcome by a vomit of tears. I wail, I stop, I continue to pack up. This will be a regular happening, I am sure.

Clare and I didn't cry together. As far as I can remember, she only allowed herself tears in my presence once in the last weeks – and they were tears of frustration. I only cried in front of her in her last moments – my last words to her. I think that was important for her to know that I had gone *beyond* what I had always been – the brother facilitating her wishes; not upsetting the energy of the room; not bringing his own sheet music to her recital.

She had carefully demarcated our relationship in this patch of time we were sharing; tried to keep it as 'clean' as possible, as the true nature of what was happening was just too 'messy'. She was always very organized.

I am finding myself drawn back to Clare's flat (I am writing this there). It will be hard to break the rhythm that we have all had over these weeks – that Dad is down the road not really able to come home for more than a few minutes at a time as he's looking after Aunty Bobs.

I don't know how many of you know the family name she had: Aunty Bobs, Aunty B. And I can't really remember how it came about – me starting to call her Bobs – a derivation, I think, of the Hungarian word for baby, *baba*. Maybe she was called that by some of our Hungarian relatives as a child. No idea. Anyway, from the moment that Gaia could speak, Clare was Aunty Bobs. And I always called her that as well – Dr Phil utterly confused on his first visit when I kept addressing her as Bobs, Bobsie or Aunty B.

I will save for another posting writing about the fourth member of our family – our son, Gaia's brother Tindy. Aunty B was an incredibly powerful force in his life, and he in hers. Their story will be told at a later time.

This has been a bit of a ramble. My thoughts are all over the place – not so surprising, really.

To finish: Grably the cat is in heaven at his new home at Ms Clarke's. I have had all the medical kit taken away by Medequip. The radio is constantly playing in Clare's bedroom – an eighties' music radio station. Scented candles lit whenever I'm here. Now I have to try to disentangle myself from this place that has been my home for the last months, reconnect with my family and the wider world. It will be hard – the bungee cord keeps pulling me back: this flat, I think, representing a simplicity, a clarity of purpose that is now gone. The world has become large again and I have to step back into it.

And all that is left is to celebrate my glorious girls still with me, Emma and Gaia. And my other glorious girl, still with me but in a different way, Aunty B.

Love to all and profound thanks for all your words, in so many different forms, over the last days.

Recurring themes

25 SEPTEMBER 2016

The universe is gently chiding me for bringing my sheet music to someone else's recital. This, more than anything else over the last weeks, has been the recurring theme, and the lesson that I will take away as homework, and have to learn. Eventually.

Don't view another person's choices from your perspective – judging them by the choices you have made. (Goodness me – this sounds a bit biblical, doesn't it?)

Oddly, it *is* something I learned long ago in my work as an actor – not to bring personal morality to bear when playing a role. Don't judge your character, just play them.

I know that this is a common trait in us humans: the terrible *looking down one's nose* at others . . .

Married couples at cohabiting ones.

Couples with kids at couples who decided not to have kids.

Couples at singletons . . .

Singletons, and single aunts in particular, are incredibly powerful beings in kids' lives – so important to have someone in your parents' generation who aren't parents themselves – the 'rogue aunt'. As an aunt and a godmother, Clare was a consummate professional: always remembered birthdays, always available for fun times, for trips, for holidays. And, in our set-up, Gaia's roommate on so many of our excellent adventures. She was a powerful free-moving spirit in so many lives – both young lives, and lives lived alongside her for all those years. Not weighty, not anchored by having children of her own, but interconnected to so many children, so many families, so many friends.

And not wanting to embark on *that* kind of love meant that the love wasn't at risk. All of us who have loved, and lost *that* way, know that the opposite of *that* love isn't hate. It's indifference (eventually – after the pain and the anger have subsided). And Clare never had to face that indifference.

Claire – the sister of my old friend, Simon, who drowned all those years ago – was a close friend of my sister as well. In a recent email, she wrote very cogently about this: '*She touched so many lives . . . she will be remembered with love – a love that will last longer perhaps than "that kind of love".*'

And an odd aligning of sentiments from another dear mate writing about a whole other friend of hers: '*It makes me think that love, real love, is more about the constant friends in my life.*'

Who am I to judge the *type* of love that Clare gave? And the *type* that she received?

Love is love is love is love. We all give and receive it in myriad ways: healthy, unhealthy; successful, unsuccessful; affirming, debilitating.

Another recurring theme of these writings over the last weeks is the power of the 'moment' – and the realization that that's all we have. A celebration of the ephemeral, I suppose.

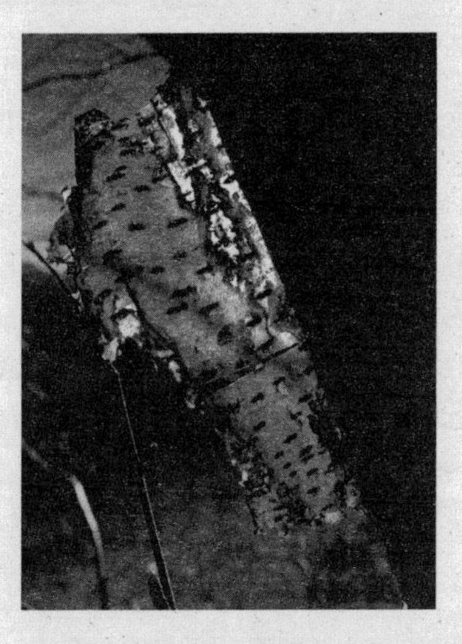

This is on the path up from our family cottage on the west coast of Scotland. A patch of wild, rough hillside, and a walk I've done probably hundreds of times. But I was stopped in my tracks on 14 February – Valentine's Day – this year. This photo is of a piece of peeling silver birch bark; the sun at just the right angle; me approaching at just the right time from just the right direction... thinking there was gold leaf on the tree. And only a minute after I'd first seen it, it was over. I'd never seen it before. And I've never seen it again.

The combination of all these disparate things aligning, just for me, just for that brief moment, giving me an enormous surge of happiness, filling me with joy and wonder and then the moment ends.

Loss is an essential part of this joy and wonder – the beauty of the Ephemeral.

And by witnessing, marking and celebrating these fleeting moments, we are both celebrating their happening and mourning their loss.

We pass by the permanent things on our journey through life without a second glance (or, if we are able, we see them again, as if for the first time, through the eyes of our small, toddling children, and hopefully share their wonderment). I always banged on about the finite nature of things bringing us the joy of the thing – would we still enjoy eating this particular slice of cake as much if we knew that this cake was everlasting? That we could have this identical slice whenever we wanted it until the end of our days? We would soon stop eating the cake... we love it because we know it's going to stop.

I am still letting the last weeks filter through me. They may filter through for the rest of my days. I don't know. And if they did, that would be fine – I think this patch of time, this loss, I will carry with me always. It will find its place within me, it will permeate, fill some gaps, make me who I am.

All I know is the incredible potency of the fleeting moments that Clare and I shared over this time. And alongside this, I know, is the desire to be able to conjure up the memory of my sister as the vibrant, powerful, funny, gorgeous, able person she was *before* all this hit her. This last week I have been clearing through her study; going through all the papers, files, boxes – a few hours ago I pulled stuff out of an envelope and had the wind knocked out of me. By this unbelievable beauty that is my sister:

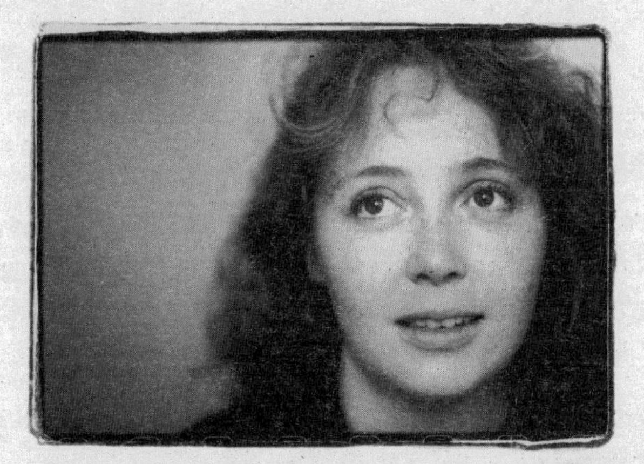

Taken by Rose, the same day as the photo recently posted of Clare with her hand over my eyes

People die. The love, the joy, the wonder does not die. The ephemeral nature of our existence creates this power, and we keep the joy of the fleeting touch within us, and carry it with us for the rest of our journey. I hope so, anyway.

And as I wrote some time ago – whatever Clare was made up of will soon go out into the universe again, to become part of something quite other, as we are just the short-term guardians of what forms us physically.

We are the embodiment of the ephemeral built of the eternal.

Love to all.

Funeral

29 SEPTEMBER 2016

Clare will be cremated tomorrow – Friday 30 September at 3.30 p.m.

There will be only seven of us there: me, Emma, Gaia and the A-Team.

I am sure that you all understand that it would have been seven or two hundred. Nothing in between. And I didn't want to make an arbitrary 'cut-off' point. So I hope you all feel that there is a fitting equality in this.

Funerals are such horrible things. Formal things. And Clare didn't want formality.

We will all have a chance to meet up in November – talk, listen, share stories, tears, laughter, drink and dance up a storm.

I will write about the funeral at the weekend.

If I can ask that you find a quiet spot if you can between 3.30 and 4 p.m. tomorrow and send a good thought out into the universe.

Love to all.

Seven

2 OCTOBER 2016

Seven heavens, seven deadly sins, seven days in the week, seven colours in the rainbow, seven oceans, seven continents, seven layers of skin, ocean waves roll in sevens, seven holes in your head, seven dwarfs . . .

. . . and seven of us on Friday afternoon to say goodbye to Clare.

I cut a huge bunch of lavender from her garden in the morning in glorious sunshine and tied it up with the drawstring of my shorts. The shorts that I had worn non-stop for all these past weeks. They came with me to the crematorium.

The seven of us (and Tindy who is still in Vietnam) had collectively designed the send-off. Clare is not your oak-coffin-with-brass-handles sort of girl, so we chose a Disco glitter-ball coffin – seemed totally appropriate for our eighties' Disco Goddess. She was dressed in a beautiful red sari, with gorgeous high heels, covered in bangles, wearing her finest shades and scented with her favourite Chanel No 5 perfume.

Our funeral director was totally unfazed by the request for four of the girls to carry the coffin – Philippa, Rose, Em and Fiona, perfectly in step, bearing their friend in to the accompaniment of the Bee Gees' 'Night Fever'.

For the next forty-five minutes we all stood around Clare, taking it in turns to speak and to make an offering to be cremated with her. I put the bunch of lavender on the coffin to start with and then my shorts. By the end we had covered the coffin with a glorious mess of offerings. So appropriate for my sister – an aesthete, surrounding herself with beautiful clean-lined pieces of twentieth-century furniture and then completely engulfing them in huge piles of clutter. I can't remember a time when I could see the surface of her dining table . . .

Midway through our offerings I noticed out of the corner of my eye a jolt from the funeral director, sitting quietly at the back of the small chapel, when Em struck a match to light an Indian incense stick she'd placed on the coffin – there's probably a Health and Safety regulation banning naked flames in a crematorium . . .

By the end we had a glove-puppet penguin, sandals, an Indian wrap, *It's a Wonderful Life* DVD, a painting of a flower by Gaia, a carrot and a copy of the play *Waiting for Godot*, photographs of Clare, all the words that had just been shared and all the wonderful words that so many of you have written to me over the last fortnight.

And a large collection of scrunched-up tissues we had all been crying into.

Clare then left us to the strains of Gloria Gaynor's 'I Will Survive'.

My wife (who has been to a funeral or two in her time) said this was the best ever. And, although hesitant to use a word like *best* when talking about a funeral, I think she was right.

Afterwards we all went off to a private space in town and made Clare extremely proud: sharing countless numbers of very fine cocktails that Gaia had invented (including a Lavender Mojito), gorgeous wines, beautiful food, wonderful stories, much sobbing and laughter, a spot of kneeling by the loo and a very professional display of alcohol-induced passing-out.

Gaia now has four new 'rogue aunts' who will take over the responsibilities that Aunty Bobs had assumed thus far – between them I think they pretty much cover all her idiosyncrasies . . .

Esther wrote to me from Antarctica saying that they had had an amazing aurora on the day of the funeral. And this, from Emma Clarke, the next day:

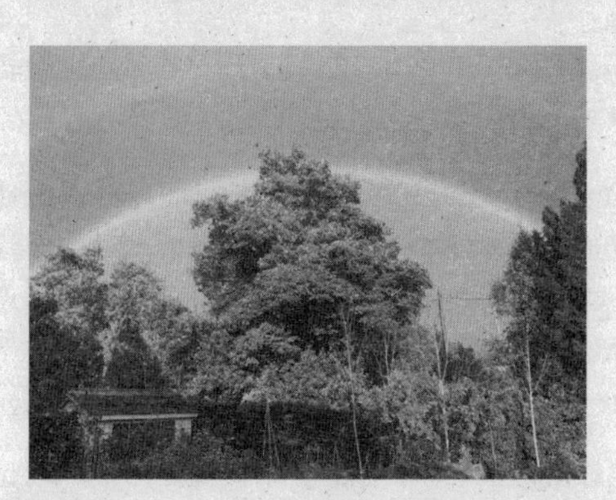

Clare's ascending in her glitter-ball and rainbows

Oh, and as Death is the joke that keeps giving... I must pass on a conversation I had on the phone last week with Clare's mortgage provider:

'You have to go into our nearest branch with the death certificate and proof that you're her executioner.'

'I'm sorry?'

'Her executioner.'

'Are you implying that I killed my sister? Do you mean her *executor*?'

Love to all.

Phantom limb syndrome

23 OCTOBER 2016

How do you start to come to terms with something that has always been there, but now isn't: like the loss of an arm or a leg? I suppose I am exhibiting a sort of phantom limb syndrome – where people who have had a limb amputated can still experience feelings in the limb as if it were still attached to their body.

I am having odd things happening with my eyesight – keep thinking there is someone just at the edge of my field of vision, but when I turn to look front on, there is nobody there. It's Clare, I am sure – forever somewhere within my view.

And my dreams are huge: most of them with my dead mum and dad in the principal cast of characters – Clare has yet to make an appearance in this part of my subconscious.

I realize that I have no touchstone to my distant past and all those memories. No second opinion (that thing that Clare was always so keen on). Nobody to jog a memory, remind me of a happening or root me in my fifty years thus far on this planet. I have no memory of life when Clare wasn't here: I am eighteen months younger than her. And she had the type of memory that could recall, in detail, what happened forty years ago – I forget what I had for breakfast this morning. I once introduced myself to someone who then quietly pointed out that we had spent the weekend together not that long before.

Are we the sum of our genetics or of our experiences, or are we a combination of both nature and nurture – and if so, is it important to remember the nurture bit? Or is that somewhere in our 'muscle memory', somewhere deep and shrouded in the firing of the synapses in our brain, somewhere beyond active recall?

I don't know. All I know now is that I have no one who was there to bear witness to me as a tiny person, pre-teen, an adolescent – both parents and only sibling gone. So, what does that mean for me? Do we need a present-day connection with where we have come from?

What forms us? Our physical selves are made from the stuff of stars (as I have explored previously in this blog) but what about the 'us' that is more mercurial, more spiritual, more indefinable?

As we get older, we hopefully unpack some stuff from the emotional rucksack that we've been carrying around for as long as we can remember – we see what is ours, which we repack and keep; what is stuff from our parents or our past that we never actively claimed, but have been carrying nevertheless, and jettison that; and what is stuff we've gathered along the way and see if it's still useful on our journey. I did a lot of unpacking and rearranging after my dad and mum died. Very good to lighten the load at that point in my early forties. But what am I carrying from the fellow traveller who was my sister? It will take time to fathom that.

Is it family that makes us who we are?

I know a little about all this because of the wonderful boy who appeared in our lives some thirteen years ago: Tindy. A refugee from Rwanda, having been kidnapped, forced into being a child soldier, escaped, and finally found himself in the UK, aged sixteen. No family, no friends, a new country and a new language. Gently, over a number of months, he became part of our family, and Gaia cannot remember a time without her brother at her side. And for Tindy, Aunty Bobs was a powerful figure: she drove him around showing him his new country; introduced him to the sea (where he rushed in fully clothed) and to his first gay couple; got him his first bike; taught him what a 'holiday' is; taught him lessons about family. And got on his case hugely about his African timekeeping and making people wait; about professionalism in an office environment; about not allowing him to think of being a porn star as a suitable profession...

Tindy is as much a part of our family as any of us. Aunty Bobs treated him as a nephew in the same way she looked on Gaia as her niece. So maybe it is not that important where we have come from, but where we are *now*; who surrounds us now, who gives us love and comfort and a sense of belonging – and not so much to do with our past loves and comforts and belonging.

These are all 'hanging thoughts' for me now. I have no answers. Maybe there are no simple answers. We are bits of everything. We are made from both the love that surrounds us and the love that has come before.

I think my favourite tree gives me the answer:

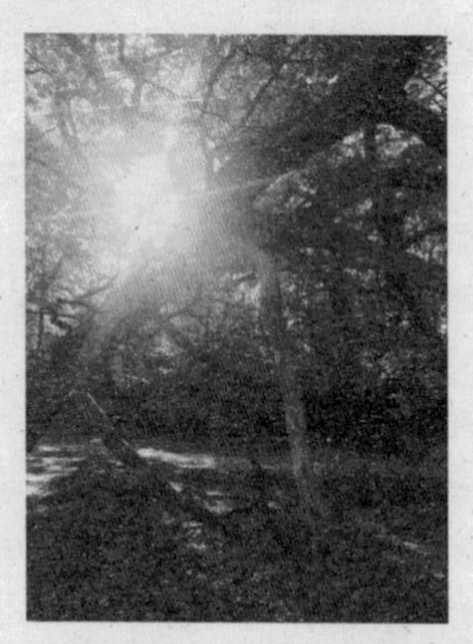

This is in a bit of woodland local to where I live and I walk past it as often as I can. I find it so incredibly moving. An ancient old oak tree, blown over in some great wind many years ago. Most of its roots sticking out of the ground, and only able to still be alive because the living part of the tree is being held up by the dead part. I find it a glorious physical manifestation of the thoughts tumbling around my head: that we truly are all propped up by those who have gone before – the living held up by the dead.

I am still spending a great deal of time in Clare's flat. Sorting, clearing, passing on, throwing away. Mostly, reasonably efficiently, but occasionally I will be thumped in the solar plexus and stopped in my tracks. Yesterday, on opening a children's book and seeing in my best ink-pen handwriting, probably aged six or seven, our two names written on the flyleaf. It was *The House at Pooh Corner* and I suppose we were Winnie-the-Pooh and Piglet – hand in hand... Clare was known by many as 'Bear', and I recently found out that Winnie was, in fact, female. So that must make me Piglet. Fair enough. Just with a more indistinctly manifested Winnie now. But she is there, nonetheless. Our relationships don't end with the ending of the person with whom we have walked hand in hand for as long as we can remember, they carry on. Just in a different form.

I feel slightly shapeless now, ungrounded, untied, somehow. I am constantly asked how I am, and that I should be doing something 'for me', something I want to do. But I have no idea of my wants. I think I need to reconnect with my body and with the earth, so I am taking myself up to the cottage in the wilds of Scotland, on my own for a week. To touch the earth, to feel the weather, to walk up in the High Places, to reconnect to my body and see how it can still serve me.

And because the jokes never stop, here's one from a letter addressed to my sister from our local council. Very angry about an unpaid direct debit of Council Tax. The overdue amount was shown and the '*Reason given by your bank: PAYER DECEASED*'.

Almost as good as a similarly computer-generated letter we received after our dad died and we had cancelled his mobile phone contract, headed, '*We're Sorry to See You Go*'.

Love to all.

Goodbye and thank you

30 NOVEMBER 2016

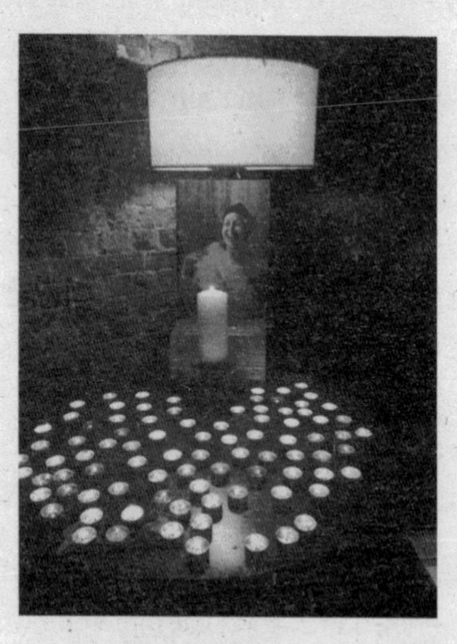

We gathered on Saturday 19 November to mourn and celebrate Clare, on what would have been her fifty-second birthday.

One hundred and twenty folk came together for the evening. Nobody there, apart from our dear friend in her box out front, knew everyone, so the evening was filled with people introducing themselves to others who they knew must be a fellow traveller of Clare's journey through life – stories told, tales learned, new friends made, tears and laughter shared.

I worked out that we had eight separate countries, four different continents, represented in the room. As a mark of the love for my sister, friends had come from mainland Europe, Africa, America and even Australia.

And befitting our 'hostess', Clare was there, at the entrance to the room, a candle burning in front of her. Everyone lit a tea-light candle from hers and created a glorious shrine. On a table next to that was a leather-bound album, where, over the evening, friends put down thoughts, stuck in photographs, jotted a few words. Some were not able to find the words at this time, but will send me their musings later and I will stick them into the book.

After a good deal of talk, the tables were cleared and two hours of pumping 1980s' Disco ensued.

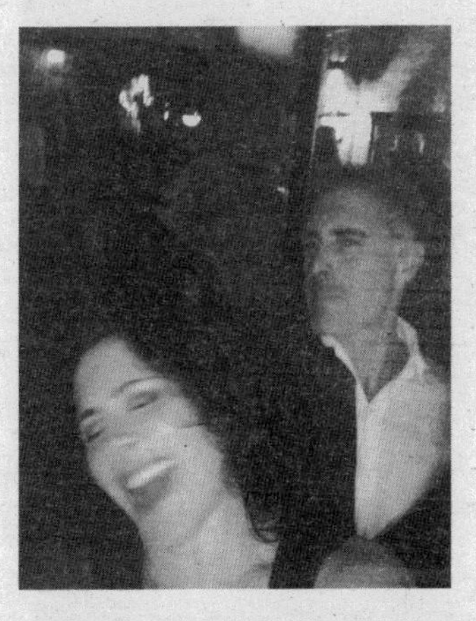

Full-on 'dad-dancing' with nobody complaining. Bliss…

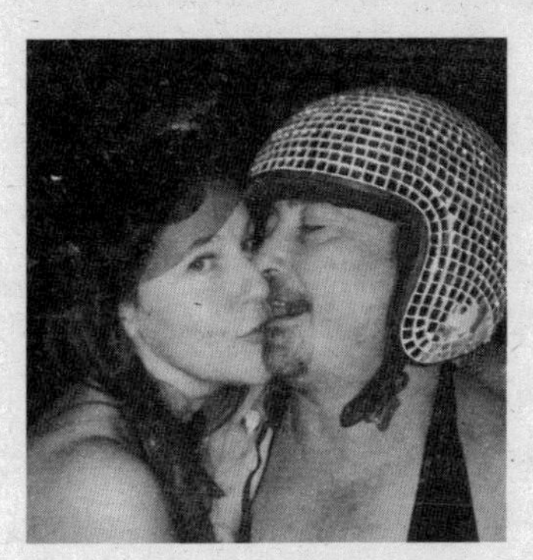

Special mention to our 'brother-from-another-mother', Warren, who flew in from Sydney: glitter-ball crash helmet, black jumpsuit and wedged shoes he had customized. Being naughty with dear Sabrina from LA

By the end of the evening, a major flurry of exchange of contact details – very appropriate for a party hosted by Clare, who always wanted people she loved to meet other people she loved. I am certain that long-lasting friendships will have started that night...

Everyone there told me just how much Clare would have loved the evening – always one for a party – and I am sure she did. We said goodbye to her in the most fitting way and the love in the room was transcendental.

And having said goodbye to her, it is time for me to stop my writings.

I took over Clare's blog primarily as a protection. For us both. As a way of not having to field phone calls, texts and emails from concerned friends. Neither of us had the strength, but knew that everyone needed to be kept abreast of where Clare was – thus I started blogging a purely arm's-length summation of the events of the day. But it soon became something else for me – it grew into something more than a collection of words typed into a machine at the end of an evening. And I won't try to deconstruct its greater meaning now, just to say that it became indispensable: a repository for my day's thoughts, feelings, frustrations, epiphanies. It soothed me to write.

I spent a number of weeks in isolation. A kind of retreat in many ways. On my own, unable to leave, mostly mute. But this time allowed thoughts to form, to gestate and to be expressed. Thoughts that I would otherwise not have had, or at least not have had the time to welcome and digest. And as I have written before – the *narrative* of these writings may have been about a Journey to Death, but I think the *theme* has been about the Act of Living. The two are the same thing, probably – can't do one well without an understanding of the other.

I have been putting off writing this last post. The final full stop ('period' for you Americans) brings with it a more-encompassing 'full stop' for me: the ceasing of collecting my thoughts, arranging them and trying to make sense of them; the laying to rest of this magnum opus – over 80,000 words now, two-thirds Clare's and a third mine – and with this comes a nagging thought that I am laying my sister to rest as a result: wrapping her up, while I move on. Nonsense, of course, but the thought remains. I know I will continue my relationship with my sister. My healthy sister. But I know I must also remember her as a cancer sufferer, and need to mark that and continue to support those who supported her.

I was honoured to be asked to open our local Marie Curie hospice – Club Med – fair last Saturday; a fundraiser with lots of stalls selling jam, hand-knitted garments, cakes and bric-a-brac. It costs £6 million a year to keep that one building up the road from us going – that's a lot of jam.

The hospice was fundamental in helping Clare stay, and eventually die, in her own home. The support they gave – from all the kit they arranged, to sitting down with Clare and gracefully and kindly explaining the situation she found herself in. I would turn up at the hospice every Friday over the last months – a sweaty mess, having just cycled up the hills, clad in my ever-more-grubby shorts and vest – to collect the prescription for Clare's weekly medications. Often I would be pulled into one of the doctors' consulting rooms, sat down and asked how I was. I was terribly British to start with – mainly just embarrassed that I was being focused on when they should have been directing all their attention on Clare, but latterly was profoundly grateful to be asked. Maybe a little too forthright when told that a bed could always be found for Clare as an inpatient if things got too much for me – replying that that would only happen over my dead body. And bless them: they gave me everything I needed to keep Clare at home.

The Macmillan Cancer Centre crowd were also wonderful. Always subsumed by the mass of patients, and thus often appointments running hours late, but always so caring. These people are at the front line in this battle. It is estimated that half of us will get cancer at some stage in our lives, and the number of people with breast cancer has nearly doubled in the last forty years. It is reaching epidemic proportions, and the fighters need our support.

Thank you all for following Clare on her journey. And I hope my taking over of writing duties was helpful to you in the last months. It has been a privilege for me.

Love to all, for the last time.

Goodbye and thank you.

Greg

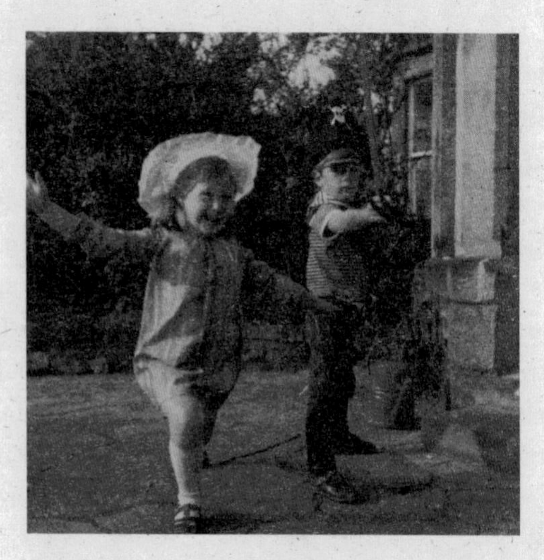